THE MISTRUTHS ABOUT DISEASE

Ethnomedicine as Applied to the Misconceptions of Health

Keith Moreno, D.N., Ph.D.

THE MISTRUTHS ABOUT DISEASE: Ethnomedicine as Applied to the Misconceptions of Health

ISBN9781484152881

Disclaimer

The information in this book is not intended to replace the services of trained, medical professionals. Neither is it intended to be a substitute for medical advice. The reader is advised to consult with his/her healthcare professional in regards to matters relating to their health and matters that may require medical attention or diagnosis.

Printed in the U.S. by Createspace

This composition is dedicated to the late *Deacon Charles Alexander Brown, Sr.*, my daughter - *Sanura*, and any person with cancer or a diagnosis that I ignored due to fear, social programming and/or the inability to question what you were told or to challenge what you believed. *I am different, now.*

Acknowledgments

I am not sure, if I will ever consider myself a writer. Of course, I am an author and I am intrigued by the conveyance of thoughts via word processor and/or with pen and paper. In addition, I am motivated by medical and agricultural mistruths. My journey of the human body and the things that affect the mind, body and spirit have been inundated with the most dominant garbage (degrees) and of course, the most carbonic and/or organic wisdom.

I am grateful for the woman that continuously attempts to complete me: *Ing.* Isabel Reza. I have surrendered my love to a beautiful woman, from a beautiful family, in a beautiful country.

My introduction to culture, language, strata, the art of quirofísica, teaching and healing in Mexico would not be complete without the thoughtfulness and patience of Qco. Antonio Gonzaléz and Centro Quirofisico.

In addition, I thank Qco. Leticia Ascensión Ríos Barraza and Qco. María Graciela López Olascoaga for trusting me with clients that wanted an alternative and had the courage to live without medications.

I long to share my knowledge with persons striving to become self-sufficient or better holistic health practitioners. Therefore, I am grateful for Qco. Graciela Gonzalez Castañeda, Qco. Juan Carlos Zapien Ortiz, Qco. Andrea Villaseñor Sanchez, and Sra. Martha Elena Linton González for giving me a chance to improve upon my teaching skills and the advancement of *Moreno Kemetic Bodyworks System*.

I do not know everything. I am open to learning, living and loving. For this reason, I am grateful to Qco. Yolanda Cruz Tesoro for pushing me to improve my Spanish and thereafter, introducing me to Qco. Oscar Martínez Zarate and Qco. Monserrat Martínez Cruz. I am appreciative of people that are selfless, encouraging and motivating.

I have met some beautiful beings. I am thankful for Ricardo Hernández of SerGay.org and the FADISEX foundation for pushing me to speak on matters that I would have accepted without questioning.

As I continue to grow and learn, I hope that I am blessed to meet more students such as Qco. Martha Patricia Martínez Zarate and Qco. Fabiola Torres Martínez.

I must admit that I am grateful to Professors Mwalimu Baruti and Ena Yaa of the *Akoben Institute* in Atlanta, Georgia for entertaining my calls, emails and questions. I cannot say that I would have the courage to assist some of the people that I encounter without your wisdom and encouragement.

Special thanks to Ashley Beck de Muñoz and Alicia Martínez for redirecting my use of Spanish and to Willem Reus for pushing me to be a better doctor.

Lastly, to any individual that I have medically or holistically failed, encouraged, assisted or awakened, I am extremely grateful for your patience, impatience, understanding, confusion and trust.

Preface

We know so much. We know more about how the body works than we ever did. About 100 years ago the first vitamin was discovered and it changed how we look at nutrition and health. We can, nowadays, run a blood test to see what nutrients are missing and supplement accordingly. We now 'know' that by consuming less fats and sugar we can effectively fight obesity. We can 'cure' many forms of cancer. It is truly exciting that so much more knowledge is available. But is it enough? And is it all true?

So, the question we should ask ourselves is why we are nowadays eating less sugars and fats, but still suffers more from obesity than any generation before us. Why, despite all the cures we have found, more and more people get sick. It is time to ask ourselves what we believe we know, and what we truly do know. One example: do you know what cancer truly is? Do you know what oxygen usage of the cells has to do with cancer? [1]Do you know why teeth, hair and bone can grow inside of some cancer? An Italian doctor believes that cancer is basically a fungus infection[2] and has research to back it up. But many others believe that the fungus, itself, is an effect.

As Aristotle Onassis once said, *"The more you own, the more you know you don't own"*. And likely, this is more true in these confusing days than it ever was. But we can only know so much. In these times we all need to specialize. A medical doctor needs to know so much about one specific field of expertise that he does not have time to question the knowledge presented to him. He just accepts the knowledge as if it is a fact, and will try to make you believe the knowledge is facts. The only way we can understand part of the knowledge is to rely on research of one part of the whole. But life is not made out of individual parts. We, humans, are only human as a whole. And only if you look at us as a whole, can you under-

---

[1] this is called Teratoma

[2] research done by Tullio Simoncini

stand that messing with one part is like Russian roulette to the whole. It is like using knowledge without wisdom.

Still, the general public believes that we have the most efficient health system there ever was since quite a number of people get well in their nighties (pajamas). Fact is that the USA is not even in the top 50 of the world's median age list[3]. The fact that most believe we are making such progress may be caused by the carefully planned and ongoing marketing campaign by those who gain the most out of it. We spend more money on drugs and healthcare than we ever did, but are not getting any better. How come? Is it not effective?

I believe that in short term situations, conventional healthcare is the most effective way to kill dis-ease. But one should always wonder about the cost of killing something inside. What good part also dies or is damaged? I am not saying there is no place for conventional medicine. It's just that holistic health is capable of preventing most illnesses. If you know how to nourish your body, you will have a natural resistance to most illnesses that goes far beyond the immune system.

In nature, if something is not getting the nutrients it needs, it will be taken care of. The low quality produce will not have a place and will be taken apart by nature's helpers so these helpers can make the limited nutrients available for other life that can flourish on the available nutrients. We call those helpers bacteria, yeasts, fungi, parasites, viruses and many other names. They are not there because you are drug-deficient, but because you are nutrient deficient. It is time we learn the truth that the big pharmaceutical industries don't want you to know. It is time that you get educated on what health is and how supporting health is often the opposite of poisoning the body to get rid of a disease.

---

[3] Median age list by Wikipedia 03-10-2013

This book, The Mistruths about Disease is about the truth that is hidden by people that profit on other people's illnesses. Choose to educate yourself. Choose the care that suits you. Choose health. But the only way to make a good choice is to see the whole truth; not just some part where other parts are carefully hidden or even made into mistruths.

Willem Reus, Proprietor of

RBTI.info

Table of Contents

Introduction

Love enabled me to mobilize my experiences of *ethnomedicine*, life, failure, determination and bitterness and relocate to Mexico City. I was accompanied by visions that required the notion of improving my life. I wasted very little time entertaining my fears because fear was taught publicly and socially in the United States. Indeed, I was very afraid. And as I began to meet clients in Mexico, I fought that which was so very American about me. I had addictions which prevented me from expressing my strengths and knowledge. My use of Spanish required work and my medical skills had to be utilized, if I was going to survive in a foreign land that was rapidly beginning to define itself as my new home.

My newfound associates were quite generous. They offered me medical cases that no one seemed to want. And there I was, clueless – as an Americanized African. I was thinking like the typical, egotistical physician. My pains ran deeply and my fears surfaced. I was suffering, emotionally and physically, but it was unlike homesickness or sciatica. My aches required me to be better and do more. I had to make changes that reached beyond verbalizing promises. After all, I was playing with my own health and needed to make changes.

In a recorded lecture, Dr. Phillip Valentine of the University of Kemetian Sciences stated, *"...because we don't know the nature of disease, the primary danger in disease is not the disease itself, but the treatments that we take – that we take. Disease is body generated. It is body conducted. It is over-seen by the body itself. Through the condition of disease (which is called many, various names) the body conducts a cleansing and reparative process upon itself. Disease is never...repeat...never, ever life-threatening. The only time disease becomes life-threatening is when man interferes with the divine process."*

I was seeking to walk in the shadows of Imhotep. Yet, my journey showed me just how much of America I had actually eaten, digested and assimilated of her poisons without ever ridding myself of her toxins. Regardless, I bathed in the wisdom of Afrika until something within me awakened. Besides, how could I look like an Olmec and not do what my Ancestors had designed me to do? I began to see the body as a whole opposed to the fragmented systems that modern science teaches and holistic practitioners unknowingly practice. The more I visualized the body, the more easily I envisioned my direction. I could not be a copy and paste, internet-type practitioner conducting myself like the majority of persons programmed by the disease industry when I had been raised in the *Hip Hop* culture and era. My education and experiences were too vast for me to shelve in an effort to be more aesthetic and clinical. Besides, I had every right to challenge anything that continued to cause harm. After all, Hip Hop had remade, influenced and repackaged every aspect of living.

I had made mistakes by trying to avoid making mistakes. I could not go forward because I was looking back and wondering if I would be noticed or challenged. My willingness to be humble was stifling my progress. And with my mistakes, the problems of Mexico became more apparent. I had to return to the basics of ethnomedicine and let my addiction to toxic, Eurocentric methods be reclaimed by their rightful owner.

This composition is a realistic glimpse into an organic heart and mind that has developed through my desire to treat my body as a temple opposed to a machine as the military-minded, pseudo-science of medicine would like for us to see it as. And too, this is my method of introducing my opinions to a country that has attracted my love and attention.

My youth, experience and/or inexperience will not allow me to share all that I know in this book: I do not know everything. However, my intentions are to assist persons in Mesoamerica and the Caribbean to understand that the various, conflicting treatments offered by the "disease industry" are the gateway to a life of suffering and bankruptcy. Moreover, the information which they have previously relied upon should not prevent them from receiving proper treatment or learning to live without synthetic medicaments, toxic behavior and nutrient-poor foods.

Spanish is a very direct and intense language. And I hope that what I have learned, through my miseducation, in America, will not make my mission more laborious than it needs to be because I am not a "language purist" and too, I have been warned to be concise; with an emphasis on simplicity. I am an emotional being that has been programmed, seasoned and socially engineered to be insensitive. Yet, I am moved by sounds, colors, odors, fragrances, and various vibrations. I am not the "new age" guru or some mentally sick individual that has decided to move south of the United States in order to reinvent oneself and charge exorbitant prices for modalities that will not work in any country - on any day. Some things just don't work despite extravagance, professional opinion, cost or hype.

I would be remiss, if I did not add the following: what we refer to as *health* is nothing more than a cultural language and interpretation. In this book, I will share information that substantiates the fact that medical data is based on melanin via the biochemical results of Europeans or melanin recessive beings. Sadly, this may be difficult to fathom, in Mexico, due to the fact that the presence of *classism* is a means of concealing the intentions of the privileged and the fact that classism, like racism, is socially constructed. However, racism — as in the United States - makes cultural intentions more blatant through the use of provisions or services intended for a particular people of unwarranted privilege while unapologetically denying others based on race, color or social status.

It is my wish - that this information motivates the reader to discover more facts about health and substances that complicate the process of living. Healing is not as complicated as the politicians, food corporations, medical institutions, health gurus, pharmaceutical companies and money-starved farmers have made it to appear. This statement, by no means, excuses the behavior and greed of poorly trained persons that have taken a position of selling anything that is not regulated by the government as holistic, natural, useful and/or effective.

With the recent inauguration of the current president of Mexico - whom the working class folks do not seemingly desire - it is appropriate that I speak and write in a tone that is indicative of my Ancestors and African health wisdom. Nowhere in this world is politics the answer for people that are capable of thinking and acting upon their thoughts.

By no means, do I wish to express an air of superiority based on melanin dominance because African historical ignorance cannot be changed with one composition or my infinitesimal, American education. Nonetheless, people are dying. A number of people are being poorly cared for and/or misdiagnosed, while others are being killed iatrogenically. And every government continues the unacceptable behavior of ignoring its duties as it maintains records of statistics that serve as guidelines for funds that will never be used for the betterment of the peoples' health or the comfort of the people that precede government.

Lastly, a many people attempt to convince the world that melanin is not a considerable, scientific factor. Sadly, some of these individuals are melanin dominant. The misunderstanding and misappropriation of the African science and art of healing has led the masses to believe that modern medicine is a science. Therefore, the strategies that have been planned and carried out as propaganda, misinformation, disinformation, cultural bias, racism and targeted neglect have been accepted without the curiosity or scrutiny of the people. It is time that the dependence and acceptance of polished ignorance undergo the challenges of anyone who loves someone.

Ch 1 Theories and Dis-ease

The word "science", alone, can give creditability to an article, report, study or opinion. People immediately assume that the mention of science is accompanied by facts. However, science in medicine - as we know it today - has been misguided by the European healing art or practice commonly referred to as "medicine".

As a melanin dominant being, I must recognize the relationship between all things in Nature. Of course, I accept the notion that all life and matter was created for a specific purpose and/or a divine reason. Certainly, all matter in Nature originated from a divine source. So, degrees and associations cannot establish my potential to utilize the overlooked importance of melanin, light, rhythm, and the vastness of the art/science of ethnomedicine.

The purpose of research is to discover the science or art of a subject in order to uncover the facts. The ignorance of the "disease industry" has permitted melanin recessive individuals to fragment the conceptualized, organic, African science of healing. Ethnomedicine uses functional, holistic research that was practiced before the ancient texts (revealed as papyri) were written. Therefore, those with money are afforded the best of research and experimentation while the disenfranchised are taxed and used as guinea pigs under the guise of "medical assistance". Neither party is at an advantage because the billions of dollars used to find what pre-historical genius recorded are merely used as justification to empower and divide, economically.

Despite one's true admiration of Greek philosophy, it was not an independently engendered invention. Truthfully, the intellect of the Greeks was nothing more than stolen intelligence from the African Mystery Systems from the Kemetic school of thought that was repackaged and accredited to a small group of pilfering Greek intellectuals. Moreover, the Greeks inconveniently located the school of Alexandria in Africa. It is crystal clear that the Greeks were learning from the Africans despite what one may think due to slanderous media reports and the treacherous intentions of greedy invaders. Be it, cultural bias, logic or racial bigotry, the global contributions of Africa should no longer be denied or white-washed. Neither medicine, astrology, mathematics, philosophy nor world history begins with the Greeks. And more importantly, Western civilizations would not be as advanced as they are without the contributions of Africa or Eastern contributions.

The idea of exalting Hippocrates as the "Father of Medicine" goes hand-in-hand with the concept of giving other Greek philosophers titles and credit for academic and scientific works that they did not deserve to have attributed to them. Nonetheless, the medical and anatomical knowledge of Africans had preceded the Greeks by no less than 3500 years. Such practices as the setting of fractures and pulse taking were being performed thousands of years before the Greeks found the courage to take the title as thieves of intellectual property belonging to Africans. In keeping with the tradition of white supremacy, the proof of African intelligence is named after the alleged founders of the papyri whom were not African.

Undoubtedly, sickness goes beyond the physical aspect because the dishonorable method of documenting historical acts is clearly rooted in racism that has prompted, justified and sustained the enslavement of the African continent and melanin dominant beings, globally. Regardless, the intentional falsification of African contributions cannot remain buried under lies for purposes of enhancing racial superiority of melanin recessive beings. And in terms of setting the record straight, Egypt should not be isolated from the greater part of Africa and offered as lineage for beings, with lesser melanin, that give reason to cultural scientists and racists to share a link to the Mother of Civilization. Furthermore, Egyptian contributions should not be viewed as the pinnacle or only contributions made by Africa or Africans.

In brief, much of what is considered to be modern medicine is nothing more than the practice of superstitions, ignorance, scientific mythology, guesswork and theories. Ironically, the modalities associated with naturopathic and homeopathic physicians and chiropractors are seen as quackery. Due to the plagues in London during the mid 1300s until the latter part of the 1600s (1348 Black Death and 1665 Great Plague), the plague doctors wore masks that resembled the beaks of ducks. As quiet as it is kept, the masks were modeled after the masks of African medicine men that used medical protective masks filled with aromatic purification herbs to maintain their health in Africa. Initially, the violence and art of self-preservation of the European surfaced and the doctors thought to be less-than-scientific were labeled as "quacks". Today, it is easy to be labeled as such. So, holistic practitioners work hard to avoid being stigmatized by the medical community.

Theoretical Views

Disease has always fascinated arrogant, ignorant scientists. The idea of said professionals ignoring the facts was mostly due to the inability to see outside of religious dogma. In their search for the cause of illnesses, with the intentions of correcting the illnesses, their level of comprehension was limited to world in which they had been exposed. To this day, theories are used to explain the various methods of healing. Centuries and even, decades ago, it was difficult to get people to think any differently than the majority believed. Today – things are not any different. It is seemingly more difficult for people to think or use cognitive skills without the persuasion of the media or government.

There are a many theories, but the Greeks deserve honorable mention, despite their undeserving recognition, because their theory was the "humoral theory". It was believed and practiced until the late 18th century. They believed the body was composed of four basic humors (fluids). The Greeks thought they could purge, leech and bleed an individual in an effort to heal them, even if it meant killing them in the process.

Humor	Season	Qualities
Blood	Spring	**Warm/Moist**
Yellow Bile	Summer	**Warm/Dry**
Black Bile	Autumn	**Cold/Dry**
Phlegm	Winter	**Cold/Moist**

The Greek geniuses actually thought that if the aforementioned humors passed through the body in the correct proportions, the individual was in good "humor". The idea of these humors presenting themselves in a deficiency or excess meant that the person was experiencing an imbalance or disease. Of course, the physician had to make a determination of the humoral imbalance based on the appearance of the vomit, excreta (feces) or mucus that was discharged during the illness.

The Greek physicians believed that the balance of the humors affected the psychological state of the person, as well. Simply put, the Greeks believed that the humors were connected to a mental state.

Mental State	Humor
Optimistic, Cheerful	Sanguine
Sluggish temperament, Unemotional, Calm	Phlegmatic
Gloomy, Sad	Melancholy
Easily angered	Choleric

The Greeks put lots of thought into this theory, in order to justify it, because each humor was associated with an anatomical reference center. Yellow bile pointed to the head, black bile suggested a problem with the spleen, phlegm was an issue with the gall bladder and blood was linked to the liver. Maintaining humoral balance involves attention to one's diet and activity in accordance with the seasons. Illnesses may be categorized by an excess of heat or cold. Naturally, the treatment of an illness under the humoral theory involves reversing an action.

The 19th century ushered in "modern medicine" and the humoral theory was abandoned. Disease is believed to be caused by an invasion of an outside source or a metabolic defect. Of course, many people are conditioned to think that an invading organism causes disease or an injury occurs and the disease enters via the damaged area. The "germ theory" is responsible for such monomorphic thinking because its foundation is based on the notion of germs attacking the body. And modern day allopathic medicine still believes in the germ theory because the practice of attacking the germ that is attacking the person, in order to restore the patient's health, continues as the premise of modern medicine and thinking.

Of all the theories in use, the "health theory" appears to be the most sensible. It is based on the idea that all disease comes from mineral deficiencies. The art of earning money under the name of medicine does not have a deficiency of theories. Anything from the colon to the pH can be used as a theory for defining the cause of disease. The health theory suggests that the body has the inherent ability to prevent sickness, if the body is well or in good health. Furthermore, said theory suggests that there are degrees of health. Despite the intentions of this theory, it must be noted that the mention of disease would not be necessary, if the body did not experience this misunderstood decline in health.

At this point, we must gain clarity about what "theory" really means. A theory can be likened to an explanation of an observation. In science, a controlled environment is preferred for the tests. Yet, the habits of scientists and doctors pressured by money makes the findings somewhat questionable. To exemplify, a large number of physicians memorize symptoms and medications and offer a diagnosis in less than 20 seconds. Basically, they guess at the problem when they do not know; the people do not believe or know that the doctor does not know. After all, the doctor can prescribe an antibiotic or pain-killer and not give the patient's condition any further thought. If the patient returns, the doctor can take another guess because they are conditioned to see their arrogance and ignorance as factual. Well, a physician's "guess" is the precursor to the first step in determining if an observation is undeniable because the first step needs to at least be an intelligent guess. This means that theory follows as the second step. Truthfully, we should concern ourselves with "facts" because theories are nothing more than unclear facts or at best, intelligent guesses.

Fast Forward to the Present

Disease means profits. Corporations, associations, scientists, lobbyists and pharmaceutical salesmen are not interested in cures for diseases. And there are a number of holistic practitioners that fashion their practices after those of allopathic physicians. They, too, attempt to kill germs.

Nonetheless, there is an overwhelming number of naturopathic physicians and holistic practitioners that believe the body is a gift from God and therefore, capable of healing itself with the proper nutrients, minerals and vitamins. Mind you, the body was designed of the same elements in the periodic table. Yet, the idea of convenience and comfort has taken a many of us away from fresh air, sunlight, proper rest, exercise, and a variety of raw fruits and vegetables. And too, the fact that a person has to take drugs (natural or synthetic) to diminish symptoms is an indication that the body is not able to heal itself due to an anatomical or biochemical malfunction. However, it is not possible to heal the body with drugs or return it to a healthy state. Again, it is not possible!

The theory that is often overlooked is that of pleomorphism. It is based on the premise that blood is not sterile. Microbiologist, Antoine Béchamps discovered microbes in the blood and referred to them as microzymas. When a person is sick, the microbes change form. In a manner of self-preservation, the microbes intelligently become disease causing in a bad environment and in a balanced environment they remain non-disease causing.

Health is complex when explained as the absence of disease. After testing urine, saliva and analyzing blood in Mexico City, it is easier to see health as the level of energy. Regardless of how people feel, they have learned to accept their health condition as normal. Most people will not notice the slightest change in their health because they expect to feel badly. The assumed energy level of the human body is between 0 and 100. At birth, a child has the energy level of seven or eight. By the time the child reaches the age of 18, the energy level should be 100. It is assumed that it will remain at 100 until the age of 80. At this time, the energy level reduces to 80. Ironically, the energy level of the average person never exceeds 35. For this reason, the health theory's assumption that there are degrees of health is seemingly a fact. If your energy level is high, the less likely you are to experience symptoms or sickness. Coincidently, one's level of energy should not be confused with desperation, discipline or the ability to perform despite knowledge of said energy level.

It is important that energy be understood because we have been told that energy cannot be destroyed or created. This is to say, that the amount of energy in the universe is constant. You cannot add to it and you cannot take from it. However, energy is being lost to the universe through the process of entropy. Moreover, it may be safe to say that life is not just energy and the lack of energy is not immediate death. Again, I am speaking of health in terms of it being seen as energy.

Naturalistic theories contributing to the causation of disease tend to continue their view of health as a state of harmony between a human being and the actual or natural environment. Humoral concepts of health and illness are widely found in Southeast Asia, India, China. Yet, in Latin America, the humoral form is recognized; but in a different form such as vitalism. Vitalism is based on the belief that disease is the result of an imbalance in the vital energies which distinguish living from non-living matter. The differences between the aforesaid theories appear to be minute, if not – semantical. For this reason, the numbers of modalities - effective and ineffective – are countless.

Despite the choice of theory, the practice of guessing at the cause of the symptoms or disease and offering a guess for the purpose of deciding how to treat the sickness is unfair to the science of healing (allopathic, naturopathic or homeopathic). Today, people utilize various types of causation in explaining an episode of illness. Therefore, the treatment may entail a variety of corresponding types of therapy. It seems logically sound that one would want to improve their health naturally - without drugs or surgery. And in terms of pain and inflammation, it is a sign that the body is working to make repairs. The inflammation and pain are designed to protect the body. And as painful as it is, it is even more agonizing to accept the fact that we do not understand our bodies enough to listen to it. We are programmed to immediately turn off the pain with drugs that cause side effects. Obviously, it is mandatory that we cease poisoning the body and permit it to do what it was designed to do.

Ch 2 Disease is not the Precursor to Death

Modern medicine is based on killing or destroying something. The patient is given medications with the idea of killing cancer, killing disease, killing blood sugars, killing tumors, killing germs and killing time - while depleting the body's natural ability to detoxify and/or repair itself. Everything is approached in a military science method opposed to medical science. The disease industry is so determined to kill something that the idea of killing the host is nothing more than a notion of romanticized collateral damage. The presence of health and the absence of noticeable pain or illness do not mean that disease is not present. Furthermore, health is not the opposite of disease. However, when the body experiences *dis*-ease or discomfort, it is a sign that the body is attempting to eliminate some form of toxicity and make necessary repairs.

The germ theory has neither been outdated nor updated because the disease industry continues to use medications to kill germs, radiation to burn out germs and surgeries to cut away germs. The public cannot imagine that disease is formed in and by the body because massive amounts of money are spent to propagate mistruths. Ironically, propaganda is very effective whether it is good or bad – true or false. Even governments are guilty of disseminating lies. Lies call for the cries of the people to demand that something be done by "Big Brother" to remedy a situation. Of course, that which is done is only a matter of reversing the damages designed and promoted by the same governmental agencies which pretend to offer assistance.

The religion of medicine has been very persuasive in conditioning its pastors, deacons and disciples to memorize signs, symptoms and prescribe drugs that do more damage than good. Lay persons argue this fact because their pains have been mitigated. Few people realize that the so-called disease has not been "killed" as intended. Yet, in the assassination process, so many healthy cells are destroyed by synthetic drugs. And once the people learn to question the god-like beings in white lab coats, with stethoscopes and/or filthy neck-ties, most will learn that what is considered a disease is nothing more than erroneous science or the body making auto-corrections.

Robert Koch established a criterion to identify the causative agent of a particular disease. If we cannot visualize health as energy or the lack thereof, we should definitely familiarize ourselves with the four postulates of this particular microbiologist that are used to determine if a given organism can cause a given disease. Primarily, the microorganism or other pathogen must be present in all cases of the disease. Secondly, the pathogen can be isolated from the diseased host and grown in pure culture. Thirdly, the pathogen from the pure culture must cause the disease when inoculated into a healthy, susceptible laboratory animal. And fourthly, the pathogen must be re-isolated from the new host and shown to be the same as the originally inoculated pathogen.

It is rather ingenious that a physician habitually diagnoses a patient in less than 20 seconds, but it is even more anti-social and arrogant that most doctors only allow a patient to speak for 12 to 18 seconds before deciding what is happening with the person that has been suffering with ailments and therefore, has more information about their body. Furthermore, most doctors become anchored to their diagnosis and refuse to believe they can be wrong. Their false sense of certainty gives the uneducated patient a sense of confidence. This thought process is the reason that the disease industry is guilty of contributing to the annual death toll. The disease industry of Mexico is not exempt from aforesaid practices because Mexico's practice of medicine is modeled after European standards and superstitions.

Hospitals are burdened and much of the staff has learned a routine that does not promote education or care. Errors and arrogance go unreported. The count of deaths due to medical errors, misdiagnosis, nosocomial infections and adverse medical reactions in Mexico has been difficult to determine, but in the U.S., alone, the reports of deaths occurring in hospitals is sickening when one considers the cost of health care, technology, education, salaries and the emphasis of germs.

WebMD dictionary defines disease as an interruption, cessation, or disorder of a body, system, or organ structure or function. If this is the best explanation of disease that the notorious disease industry can offer, death should not be as common as it is. And if Koch's postulates are so outdated that they are not used to determine infectious diseases; and do not apply to special, inexplicable retroviruses, but continue to apply to routine viruses, then the modernized disease industry should explain and publish the new criterion that serves in a galaxy in which the so-called human body is not changing. That is to say, there are no new ways of dying. In addition, there are no new ways to obtain health. The basics of life and longevity will not change and expensive healthcare will not improve one's chances of avoiding the causality of disease or untimely death when we disobey the laws of Nature.

When people dismiss the idea that their diagnosed problem was caused by germs, they then contend with the thought of having a disease because of bad luck, the absence of God in their lives or even genetics being the root cause. Consequently, these same people think that only synthetic drugs, surgeries and expensive advice are the only remedies for their ailments. Few people understand that they have not been diagnosed because they are sick. Nonetheless, they think they are sick because of the diagnosis. There is a difference. And the difference gradually tears through the fibers and foundation of a family. However, modern medical practices are not the answer to the problems of any country, community, tribe, family or individual whether they can afford to die a painful, slow, expensive death or not.

In the new age introduction of medicine, every practitioner boasts of having the cure to disease. And certainly, every practitioner has healing powers. Every article mentions the need for alkalinization and oxygenation based on the theory that diseases develop in the presence of acidic and non-oxygenated cells which are caused by bodily imbalances that are a result of malnutrition. Most theories push the sale of alkaline products like alkalinized water, pills that alkalinize water, alkaline water purifiers and alkaline supplements. Sick people that swear by the products and promise results are selling alkaline products and promising results that cannot contend with the rate and amount of processed foods and/or pharmaceuticals that are ingested on a daily basis. The popularized theories will not work for everyone and alkaline products are not beyond the most sophomoric methods of healing or poisoning. After we identify what vitamins and minerals the body lacks, we can procure the necessary enzymes, vitamins and minerals needed to reverse the complications that the body endures.

The word care comes from the Latin Word *cura* which has various meanings such as management, administration, care, concern, charge. In addition, care is defined as the provision by a physician of services related to the maintenance of health, prevention of illness, and treatment of illness or injury. Why is this word a medical term? Why does the disease industry allow doctors to claim a cure of a disease and then claim that it was in remission after the patient (another medical term) is revisited by the disease?

Despite what the world thinks of Mexico or Latin America's sanitation and hygienic practices, the leading causes of death are not associated with infectious diseases or diseases caused by fecal matter. Like the U.S., Mexico suffers from heart disease, cancer and obesity. Any and every medical association knows that the diagnosis of a chronic or fatal disease can destroy the mental, emotional and financial status of a family. Regardless, doctors are trained to be conniving and non-emotional like nothing more than mechanics charging a woman for parts her car does not need. In other words, doctors are trained to look for sickness. They do not understand health and are not trained to look for it.

As we meditate on the bigger picture, it appears as if a disease awaits us all. Even if we escape a fatal disease, a smaller disease requiring expensive treatments and medications awaits each and every person that indulges in refined foods and medications. As we consider misdiagnosis, it is frightening to entertain the thought of being told that you or a family member has a disease. Surely, the disease will take its toll on your health and you will want to give up. If you have family, they will possibly find ways to get the money; even if it means that they have to endure economic hardship. To no surprise, the treatments and medications will not cure the disease which you probably do not have. However, the use of pharmaceuticals can result in an illness. It is imperative that people learn about the functions of the body, the nature of disease and why bodies display symptoms or develop diseases.

The poor are eating poorly due to poor choices and limited finances. And the rich are eating poorly because their expensive meals are prepared by those with educations that are costly, but worthless. By trusting the government's daily requirements, food group suggestions and sanctioned foods, anyone can die a death caused by chronic disease or the results of misdiagnosis while enduring subsequent poverty. It is time that people rethink the science of eating that has been over-thought, over-processed and made into a deadly art designed for taste.

The disease industry is nothing more than a church of modern medicine. Yet, most of what is considered modern medicine is a new understanding or more of a misinterpretation of the medical annals of Africa. Science should not be confused with theory or philosophy. Pharmaceutical companies and doctors are able to prove very few things, but people believe the limited information and the prevalent mistruths. The masses have faith in the men in white. The medical field has purchased and patented words. Some words are automatically associated with religion. Belief and faith are definitely religious terms. Without these terms, the disease industry would be exposed. Regardless, science is not a necessary requirement of medicine because science seeks the truth. This truth is substantiated by proof. Today, modern medicine is a religion built on faith, myths and beliefs disguised as science.

There are a number of medical myths which societies throughout the world accept as proven truths. The disease industry pushes for legislation that forces the masses to use products that are useless for intended use, but harmful due to deception. People actually believe that midwives are not as intelligent or effective as doctors; HIV causes AIDS; condoms prevent the spread of AIDS; fluoride is safe and necessary; radiation will not destroy good cells; chiropractors are not doctors; sun-block prevents skin cancer; vaccinations are safe; HIV tests are accurate; government approved foods and medications are safe and better than herbs; mercury fillings are harmless; and mammograms reduce the rate of breast cancer. These are a few of the lies that the disease industry does not have to prove. However, the internet attracts articles everyday that attempt to discredit Nature or ridicule natural medicine. Deaths continue to add up and the medical sciences are excused and the deaths are seen as the work of God or perhaps, a body diseased beyond repair.

It is clear that the disease industry does not ever intend to uphold the Hippocratic Oath. Practitioners of the disease industry are faithfully giving treatments that cause harm and death. And too, they rely on poisonous pills to solve or calm issues they do not understand or wrongly diagnose. And despite the fact that some practitioners really do care about human life, most are simply doing as told or taught. And the majority of practitioners - be it allopathic, homeopathic, naturopathic - have a limited understanding of nutrition and nature because their aim is to be accepted by the most prestigious of all medical associations.

It would be wonderful to see the masses become more self-reliant, but the education system is not designed to unshackle the mind of anyone that is impressed with consumerism or being controlled. As consumers, we are susceptible to the advances of anyone with something to sell. The disease industry and Big Pharma are masters at marketing via word-of-mouth, print-ads, doctors and commercials. They use bad science, confidence and fear to rob families of their future or any chance at prosperity by ignoring the logical causes of disease that are more than apparent. Complicated diagnoses coupled with the use of Latin (prescriptions) and arrogance blinds the masses and causes them to trust their bodies and health to people that would rather sell drugs and surgeries. Such trust is expected to be unwavering in order for the hospitals and pharmaceutical companies to generate large sums of money while fostering the family's dependence on lucrative treatments and toxic drugs.

Herbs cannot be patented, yet. However, man will continue to challenge Nature and steal from her by synthetically duplicating her intent and genius. Surely, technicalities present a margin for theft because of duplication and poisoning, but manufacturers are not willing to put up the money to prove that an herb is medically safe because opinions claiming they are unsafe are much cheaper. Nature does not need to be validated by man. As for "disease" — there really aren't any needs for cures because the body isn't seeking any. The body heals itself when it is allowed to do so. From my perspective, toxemia and nutritional/mineral deficiencies are the best candidates for causes of disease. So, as we struggle to understand what causes the immune system to fail, we should demand of ourselves to partake in proper nutrition, physical exercise, lifestyle modification and an attitude of harmony, order, truth, balance, morality and justice.

Holistic and organic are two misused terms in the world of marketing. And some holistic practitioners are guilty of over-looking the whole being and attacking what is visible to the eye. Holism suggests the treatment of a disease without making distinctions between the organic wholes and ignoring the   feasibility of visualized units or organs and negating their existence beyond the sum of what said organ or unit is thought to be.

We are fascinated by disease because we have been conditioned to like lies. In essence, the majority of people are enthralled with the lack of responsibility associated with not being in charge or the idea of not having to think. Pimping may be easier than we think because the pimps are not necessarily sharing information about how not to be gullible, how not to be considerate, or how not to be affected by the humility or fear of the majority. Pimps are occupied with control, manipulation and illusions. Sadly, the majority of people are incapable of straddling the fence. Thus, they are being pimped, while complaining and secretly admiring the pimp or poorly pimping someone and still not finding satisfaction with their position in life. We are programmed to want more or envy what some other individual has. Unfortunately, what others supposedly have can actually be less or more. Nonetheless, it causes us to question the meaning of success, happiness, satisfaction, moderation and even, monogamy. It is part of "the game" and anybody in need of something that another entity supplies, is a player or merely a consumer.

As long as we trust governments and manufacturers, we will be viewed as victims, consumers and willing sacrifices: we have become whores for the powers that be due to our willingness to comply with their suggestions or demands without questioning our own discomfort. There are sufficient numbers to make a difference in how the masses are treated, but just as most have learned to accept pain and illness with aging, people accept chemically enhanced soils, bad foods, and poor living situations and readily adapt to bad situations. This mentality implies that if the cell doors were visible, the people would voluntarily assist the guards in closing and locking them.

Diseases are not dirty little secrets waiting to enter our bodies. The thought of organs or organisms malfunctioning due to germs or contagious diseases, as expressed by the paranoid ideation of the disease industry, is a part of an ignorance that cannot continue to grow. Our bodies are exposed to stress in various ways and Nature has designed a method that permits the body to respond in times of psychological or emotional distress.

I have emphatically stated that there is no new way to die and I am confident that the disease industry will not find any equipment or pharmaceuticals to improve upon what the human body, accompanied by the wisdom of true healers, is designed to do. It has been easier for man to accept the "Holy Trinity" than the fact that science and academics cannot fragment the human experience or simply make it "physical". African wisdom emphasizes the existence of mind, body and spirit. Undoubtedly, the wisdom of African medicine has never denied this fact. African wisdom does not recognize unforeseen incidents as accidents and attempt to bandage them. Instead, the site of damage coupled with vibrations or the absence of vibrations is seen as a warning or an indication of what is.

Since my arrival in Mexico, I have come to believe that I can improve the perception of ethnomedicine. Of course, I have learned that some individuals are so toxic that I must find ways to distract them while the body does what it is naturally designed to do. Unlike most doctors (allopathic, homeopathic, naturopathic) and egotistical persons selling natural products, I have learned that no two people are alike. I respect "life". I adore Nature. As an Afrikan, I do not fear disease and I will not make a division between mind, body and spirit. I have to visualize the mind, body and spirit as a whole.

Man cannot contend with Nature. Scientific facts can and should be questioned when it is fatal. We, now, know that a virus is a microscopic, infectious particle that is fully assembled. It is infectious because the particle produces other particles with identical appearances by virtue of its ability to enter and live on or in a cell. Yet, this explanation, alone, does nothing to alter one's confidence to challenge the intellect of mechanical logic that is applied to science, the disease industry or the doings of Big Pharma.

The Mistruths about Disease

It is very common to see people eating in Latin America because eateries are everywhere. In addition, people eat late hours due to work schedules and time needed to commute via public transportation and/or contend with the continuous traffic. Surprisingly, people - around the world - have been taught to eat constantly and undoubtedly, to feed ailments. However, when a person feels tired or sick, the body is sick and the energy is low. This can and will occur with any form of food that is not in its natural form because the body can only digest so much. And too, the most desired foods that are socially craved by the majority rarely have any energy.

When the body lacks energy, digestion is difficult. Normally, digestion of newly ingested foods is difficult because we are constantly eating and drinking. Once the body has digested food, energy is released for other things in the body. Unfortunately, the suggestions offered by culture, religion, media and government can be more   persuasive than the truth. Besides, fueling — which is about giving the body what it needs in order to ascertain that it functions well — is unknown to consumers. Most people think of sugar in the form of the insidious white powder or a candy bar, energy bar, piece of candy or maybe, an energy drink. The body's struggle to rid itself of toxins, as it fights the foreign substance, is mistaken as a burst of energy.

We eventually look for the secrets that promise longevity, beauty and youth after we have started to lose vitality and confidence. The idea of properly eating and avoiding processed foods is not important until we sense that our lifestyle is attracting pain and illness. Even more frightening is the possibility that what we eat is abbreviating our life. Today, eating is the act of consuming food for nourishment, social activity and enjoyment. It is no longer an activity designed for survival.

Preventive health is not very important because it goes against consumerism. Consumerism guarantees ignorance, profits and disease. Therefore, the degradation of minerals and vitamins in the food supply is minimized by corporations. Certainly, the disease industry does not act up or speak out because a sick consumer is a valuable patient. Magazine ads, television commercials and billboards keep our attention with meaningless, fabricated foods accompanied by chemically enhanced flavors and more shelf-life than cotton candy.

Mineral depletion and degenerative diseases should be attributed to soil depletion. Of course, refined foods are damaging the minds and bodies of people, but the long-term accumulations of poor nutrition that are recognized as cancer, diabetes, obesity, et cetera were not known before the influence of technology, mass production and chemical manipulation. The consumption of minerals and vitamins was easier to obtain without the government's decision to inaccurately "dummy proof" boxes and cans with information that consumers both read and trust wholeheartedly or possibly read and don't understand.

Farmers are evidently aware of the changes in the soil because their wealth and basic concern is in the soil. We are literally starving to death despite how much we eat. And we are eating more than we should eat. We eat before meals, while cooking meals, while waiting for meals, in between meals and after meals. From the time we awake until we are asleep, we are periodically tasting and swallowing. Unfortunately, the people that do not have food are suffering as well. It is too late to blame negligence or the ignorance of soil fertility and the misconceptions about the production of healthy crops.

Throughout Latin America, nutritional disorders are responsible for a major segment of the factors limiting the productivity of livestock. Mineral deficiencies in livestock intended for consumption by humans are demonstrated by clinical signs of diarrhea, anemia, loss of appetite, skin disorders, bone abnormalities, tetanus, low fertility, miscarriage and hair loss. Long before humans develop a habit of eating dirt, starch, cushion from pillows or any other non-nutritive substance, animals experience the Pica disorder in preparation for the slaughter. And humans are expecting to receive nourishment from animals that are diseased and dying before they sense their slaughter. Money buys opinions and there exists a portion of investigators that argue that the livestock suffer the same clinical signs even when given an adequate feed supply. This can only mean that factory farm animals are a detriment to the health of humans; even if, they are eaten in moderation.

Good soil consists of a good mineral supply and naturally produces crops with a profound resistance to disease and insects. Of course, adding nitrogen, phosphorous and potassium will not prevent malnutrition or nutrient-poor produce. It must be known that produce from nutrient-dense soil does not rot. Instead, it dehydrates. Nutrient-poor produce rots. Yet, the world is learning to live from foods that barely curb hunger pains. Still, said foods are trusted to nourish and heal the body. Eventually, the farmers that make a living by planting and selling only one crop will realize that monoculture has its disadvantages. As the people get sicker and the soil further deteriorates, it is better to employ multi-cropping and crop rotation systems. The concept of   multi-cropping uses one crop to replace a crop requiring different nutrients. In addition, multi-cropping is good because the various crops protect each other from insects and disease.

The United States of America is considered to be on the top end of the evolution of countries. This means that it is a first world country. Sure, the lights can still go out at the Super Bowl, 15% of the population can be impoverished, millions can be found without a home and hundreds of thousands of people can die from mistakes caused by doctors, hospitals and medications. And this is the country that other countries wish to be replicas of? Nonetheless, America has issues. I am inclined to think that America did not knowingly and willingly create these problems for herself. She has so many resources and no idea of how to police herself as she gains enthusiasm about her self-appointed position as the *Guardian Angel of the World*.

Attractive packaging coupled with clever marketing by the organic industry has lead people to believe that "organic" is safe, clean, better tasting, nutritious and locally grown. And let's not forget how expensive it is, because people are willing to pay for value. Truthfully, animals and big food corporations are the greatest benefactors of the organic trend. The people should not have to pay for foods to be grown without poisons. And using land to raise livestock should not take precedence over the use of land to grow produce.

Dr. Keith Moreno

Perception of Change

Latin Americans have an advantage over the United States because the people have naturally adopted a life that embraces traditional foods, family cohesion, an eco-friendly lifestyle and bartering. In addition, alternative or natural medicine is appreciated. There doesn't need to be a rush for change because the aforementioned qualities no longer exist in the U.S. What was once perceived as abnormal is now a normal and accepted part of society despite the increase of decadence.

The thought of abnormalities brings to mind the modalities that holistic practitioners use for financial gain. Admittedly, some methods are as useless as some of the experiences and educations of the practitioners. Furthermore, it is an obvious fact that some practitioners lack the capacity to heal. Some practitioners argue that the disease industry is killing people. However, large percentages prescribe herbs as if they were synthetic drugs; sell illicitly procured pharmaceuticals; and perform questionable practices. The need to earn money and the desire for prestige has corrupted the purity of nature and the science and art of healing.

The allopathic belief system recognizes disease and symptoms as all in the same. This is the reason that a so-called "cold" is assumed to be healed when the cough, sneezing, headache or sniffle is no longer an apparent issue or sign. If the truth be told, the elimination of a symptom is likened to the suppression of a symptom. The root cause must be identified and eliminated or one can expect an eventual emergence that appears in a form that is more chronic and convincing. This is not an issue because the masses have been programmed to take a pill for any pain and every symptom.

The Food

Mexico has an abundance of fresh produce. Whereas, the majority of food in the U.S. is shipped, gassed, waxed and warehoused. Mexico is the second fattest country in the world. But with an introduction of more "fresh" foods and an understanding of variety, Mexico could be much healthier. However, the meal base consisting of traditional chopped meat and tortillas are religiously consumed each day. This has to be addressed and studied.

Granted, vegetarianism is not very popular in Mexico. Of course, vegetarian restaurants do exist in the country of meat and bread. Yet, enforcing a meat-free diet is difficult for anyone who is convinced that protein is important. What is more difficult to conceive is the idea that protein can only be obtained from meat. Meat is just as addictive as nutrient-poor foods that people entertain themselves with from the time they awake until they fall asleep. Ironically, some people awake during the night just to eat more food. In terms of energy that is often mistaken as health, some meats will reduce an individual's level of energy more quickly than others.

The Joys of Meat

It is pointless to argue the preservation of animals and then turn a blind-eye to the violence caused by the war-on-drugs, wrongful incarceration, wear a leather jacket with a mink collar, attend a dog fight or horse race, eat an egg, drink a milkshake or never question authority. People will always eat meat. Meat infected with feces, meat from animals with diseases, meat frightened before slaughter and meat that knew from its first breath that it was destined for death. Meat, ignorance and fear will never be in demand because there will always be an abundant and prevalent supply.

In terms of eating meat, the consumer has been conditioned to believe that meat is a necessity. Of course, there are a number of sources from which to procure meat. Manufacturers offer free-range, bred free-range, organic and factory-farmed meat. The people want meat and the people will get meat. Meat, milk, cheese and eggs are in demand. So, animals are tasked with sacrificing their lives to ascertain that the people get the diseases that the government refuses to make them aware of. The China Study proved that by increasing dietary animal protein in the presence of a carcinogen increased the enzyme activity that then allowed that carcinogen to transform into a dangerous metabolite with the potential to bind onto and mutate DNA. To avoid a tone of political vegetarianism, it is easier to assume that the animals will be dispatched to death for the convenience and enjoyment of consumers than to argue the reasons to avoid the consumption of animals and animal-byproducts. Furthermore, The China Study illustrated that low protein diets reduced tumors by having less carcinogens enter the cell and therefore, reducing the multiplication rate of cancer cells.

Mexico is a god-fearing, religious country. For this reason, it is only fair that the public know what is considered clean or unclean meat according to the scriptures. Of course, each denomination and religion has its own interpretation of the Bible and other scriptures. Moreover, people are free to eat as they wish and of course, what they desire...in ignorance or in their miseducated denial. Based on melanin (not pigmentation), the more melanin dominant being should eat a more alkaline, carbohydrate type of diet opposed to an acidic, meat type diet designed and approved for melanin recessive beings.

Clean and Unclean Animals

11th chapter of Leviticus contains laws regarding eating animals.

Now the LORD spoke to Moses and Aaron, saying to them, *"Speak to the children of Israel, saying, these are the animals which you may eat among all the animals that are on the earth: Among the animals, whatever divides the hoof, having cloven hooves and chewing the cud; that you may eat. Nevertheless, these you shall not eat among those that chew the cud or those that have cloven hooves: the camel, because it chews the cud but does not have cloven hooves, is unclean to you; the rock hyrax (small, robust ,furry animal), because it chews the cud but does not have cloven hooves, is unclean to you; the hare, because it chews the cud but does not have cloven hooves, is unclean to you; and the swine, though it divides the hoof, having cloven hooves, yet does not chew the cud, is unclean to you. Their flesh you shall not eat, and their carcasses you shall not touch. They are unclean to you."*

Among the animals, whatever divides the hoof, having cloven hooves and chewing the cud; that you may eat: The rule was and is... simple. If an animal has a divided hoof (not a single hoof like a horse), and chews its cud, it could not be eaten.

The following can be eaten: **Antelope, Beef (Domesticated Cattle), Buffalo, Deer, Goat, Lamb, Roebuck and Sheep.**

These you shall not eat among those that chew the cud or those that have cloven hooves: For example, the camel, the rock hyrax, and the rabbit all chew the cud, but do not have divided hooves - instead, they have paws - they are considered non-kosher. Chewing the Cud means to chew food, swallow it and then brings it up to chew again. They then swallow the food into another stomach.

There are other scriptures that speak of comestible meats and warn of eating detestable things and avoiding the consumption of meat that you find dead. However, the references are for individuals that depend on meat while their body is weak, malnourished and/or healing.

And the swine, though it divides the hoof, having cloven hooves, yet does not chew the cud, is unclean to you: Additionally, the swine has a divided hoof, but it does not chew the cud - so it is considered non-kosher.

Their flesh you shall not eat and their carcasses you shall not touch: If an animal was considered unclean, one obviously could not eat it. Yet additionally, one could not touch an unclean animal, whether living or dead.

No matter what you think about pigs, they are filthy animals. They are considered scavengers and were created to eliminate waste. They eat anything; garbage, bugs, anything lying around, insects, feces, dead carcasses (human or of dead, sick animals).

China is the largest producer of pigs. The Center for Disease Control and Prevention in the U.S. has stated that more than 100 viruses come to the United States each year from China through pigs. Pork is loaded with toxins because the pig digests meat rather quickly and it does not have sweat glands. The toxins are not eliminated. They are stored in the fatty tissues and readily available, despite cooking temperatures, when prepared for consumption. Moreover, the pig carries several parasites. Unfortunately, some of the parasites cannot be destroyed by cooking. Trichinellosis and trichinosis is the biggest concern with eating pork because the trichinella worm makes its home in the muscles of the pig.

The pig is the primary carrier of the following diseases:

- Hepatitis E Virus

- Nipah Virus

- Taenia Solia tapeworm

- Menangle Virus

- Porcine Reproductive and Respiratory Syndrome (PRRS)

Water Animals That May Be Eaten

"These you may eat of all that are in the water: whatever in the water has fins and scales, whether in the seas or in the rivers; that you may eat. But all in the seas or in the rivers that do not have fins and scales, all that move in the water or any living thing which is in the water, they are an abomination to you. They shall be an abomination to you; you shall not eat their flesh, but you shall regard their carcasses as an abomination. Whatever in the water does not have fins or scales; that shall be an abomination to you."

These you may eat of all that are in the water: The rule remains simple: Any water creature having both fins and scales is considered kosher and can be eaten.

Whatever in the water has fins and scales, whether in the seas or in the rivers; that you may eat: On this principle, most fishes were considered clean - except a fish like the catfish, which has no scales. Shellfish are unclean, because clams, crabs, oysters, and lobster all do not have fins and scales.

Birds/Fowl That May Be Eaten

"And these you shall regard as an abomination among the birds; they shall not be eaten, they are an abomination: the eagle, the vulture, the buzzard, the kite, and the falcon after its kind; every raven after its kind, the ostrich, the short-eared owl, the sea gull, and the hawk after its kind; the little owl,

the fisher owl, and the screech owl; the white owl, the jackdaw, and the carrion vulture; the stork, the heron after its kind, the hoopoe, and the bat."

These you shall regard as an abomination among the birds: There is no rule given to determine if a bird is clean or unclean. However, we should avoid predators and scavengers because they are unclean.

The following are clean according to Biblical law: Chicken, Dove, Peafowl, Pheasant, Pigeon, Quail and Turkey.

Insects That May Be Eaten

"All flying insects that creep on all fours shall be an abomination to you. Yet these you may eat of every flying insect that creeps on all fours: those which have jointed legs above their feet with which to leap on the earth. These you may eat: the locust after its kind, the destroying locust after its kind, the cricket after its kind, and the grasshopper after its kind. But all other flying insects which have four feet shall be an abomination to you."

All flying insects that creep on all fours shall be an abomination to you: Among insects, any creeping insect was non-kosher. Yet, if there is a flying insect with legs jointed above their feet, these could be eaten. Good examples of kosher insects are the locust, the cricket and the grasshopper. Insect consumption can be confusing due to the scientific meanings of Hexapoda, Myriapoda, and Arachnoidea.

We are given the choices of eating to survive and eating to live. One decision focuses on enjoyment and one requires conscious effort. We can claim to be busy or not know how to cook, but as our health declines the ability to earn a living naturally diminishes. And regardless of what we think of fast food, it is eaten by millions of people every day. People don't think about high calorie content or poor quality when they are hungry or just out to enjoy a meal that they could have gone without. Food fills voids. Food is comforting to the minds of food junkies as it is being consumed. Food is addictive! Food is the drug that food pushers don't want you to discover. The stuff we've come to call "food" is diminishing our longevity and poisoning any possibility of a fountain of youth.

Unlike the U.S., fast food in Mexico is over-priced and the workers are not in a rush to offer fast service. Ironically, in the U.S. people demand that meals come quickly because they assume fast food means "speed and efficiency of service" and undoubtedly, most people are in a hurry. Fortunately, the lower income families of Mexico are not as easily threatened with obesity, high cholesterol, or the consumption of plastics and oils that are provided through poisonous franchises with no real indication of nutrition. However, a large percentage of impoverished Mexicans are affected by *Gansitos* and *Coca Cola*. Moreover, the average food chains popularized in the U.S. are seemingly eateries for the middle-class of Mexico. Ironically, the desired foods do not represent the local cuisine.

Regardless of where you live, you have been given more lies about food than you can imagine. For example - it is a myth, if not a lie, that we evolved through periods of feast and famine to be very good at holding onto fat. Just who is the "we" that science speaks of? Such talk cannot speak to melanin dominant beings. Fat gain is due to excessive insulin levels caused by high dietary, refined carbohydrate intake. It is a sign that something in the body is going wrong. It is not a healthy adaptation. Restricting calories with a low fat/high carbohydrate diet just makes you hungrier and more lethargic. It even slows your metabolic rate. Weight-loss is only maintained if the person stays on a semi-starvation diet forever or implements fasting into their life. Insulin is the overall fuel control for humans. High insulin levels cause the body to store fat and stops the body from using fat as fuel. This means that high carbohydrate foods make you put on more fat and leave you still feeling very hungry and unsatisfied. And lastly, people have different insulin secretory responses. Even if insulin secretion is slightly off, weight gain can still occur.

It is important that we not see a calorie as a calorie or adopt an attitude of calories in and calories out. To even call it a heat unit and not be able to burn it away is useless. Furthermore, low-calorie diets lack nutrients. We have to begin to think and question the manufacturers of our food and pharmaceuticals, if we are not going to use what nature has provided.

Additional Foods to Avoid Once You Experience Changes in Health or Energy Levels

- Coffee, sodas, energy drinks and caffeinated water.

- Tea (contains tannin)

- Sea Salt

- Pasteurized, anti-oxidant, super fruit juices with artificial sweeteners and/or high fructose corn syrup.

- Red meat (Beef, veal, lamb, venison, pork, goat, rabbit and Buffalo). Any meats derived from mammals are considered to be red meats.

- Barbacao (whole sheep/meats slow grilled over open fire)

- Cabeza (roasted head of cow)

- Carne Asada

- Lengua (tongue of cow)

- Machaca (shredded beef)

- Picadillos

- Sesos (beef brains)

- Tripas/Machitos

• White meat refers to any light-colored meat like fish, seafood, and poultry. However, it includes any of the meats that are considered to be less fatty in comparison with red meats. The term white meat comes from the fact that the meat of chicken is white in color. The most popular of white meats are animal proteins derived from birds such as chicken, turkey, duck, goose and quail. Fish (catfish, tuna, mahi-mahi, mackerel, and eel), reptiles (alligator, snake), amphibians (frogs' legs), crustaceans (lobster, shrimp, crab, and crawfish) or bivalves (oysters, clams, scallops, escargot and mussels) should also be avoided.

• Al Pastor

• Carnitas

• Chicharrones

• Pollo Asada

• Pasta

• White rice

• Tortillas

• Bread. Substitute leafy greens for bread if you want to

enjoy a healthy sandwich.

• Dairy. This means low-fat products, cheese, milk-based

yogurt, whey products, and anything that contains

casein (glue made from milk). This includes goat milk

products.

• Gelatins made from animal by-products.

• Eggs

- Chocolate (contains tannin)

- Popcorn (because the hulls stick to the colon)

- Nutmeg

- Hard seeded fruit (strawberries, raspberries, blackberries).

- Corn syrup

- Agave (contains high fructose corn syrup)

- Cassava

The following foods should only be eaten in **moderation** because they cause a loss of energy. Again, health is about energy.

- White sugar. If you must sweeten food, use stevia, dates, Raw cane sugar or coconut sugar.

- White flour

- Whole grain flour. If you must eat white flour or whole grain flour, eat in moderation and too, as a mixture of half whole grain and half white flour.

- Salt

- White potatoes (calcium oxide is difficult to digest).

Camote, sweet potato, and yams are okay to eat.

- Butter

- Margarine (with transfat)

- Milk (whole, 2%, low fat, 1%, etc)

- Soy Milk

- Yogurt. Vegetarian (non-animal gelatin) is ok.

- Black pepper

- White pepper

Food on the Brain

We have been taught to view the body as a machine. However, the human body is more complex and mysterious than any machine that man fashions or programs. We have so much to learn about the body. Actually, machines are modeled after the human body. Consequently, man designs and fabricates machines; not vice versa.

The time and money put into drugs and machinery may never compare to the intricacies of creation. Not a minute of the day is exempt from chemical reactions that take place throughout every cell or tissue of the body. Of course, food supports these chemical reactions. Once we understand the importance of food and the body, we will see that the biochemical reactions involve breaking down larger molecules into smaller molecules, building something from the food, or converting something into something. There is so much chemistry occurring in the body. Add the brain to the chemistry and we have more than 10 billion nerve cells, trillions of connections and billions of nerve pathways. So, the complex machine has a remarkable computer. The Greeks once believed that the brain was a cooling system because of the cavities in it that were filled with fluids. Nevertheless, we can agree that the brain is a chemical factory.

It is imperative that we understand the Krebs Cycle, as well. Without it, we would not be able to generate efficient energy from the carbohydrate content of your food. Carbohydrates are available from two sources: simple and complex carbohydrate foods; or more appropriately, foodstuffs such as cereals, grains, fats and oils derived from animal and vegetable by-products. They are also available from proteins, which are composed of amino acids at the head of the molecule with a carbohydrate tail.

Carbohydrate by definition contain only carbon, hydrogen and oxygen molecules. Plus, they can be converted to glucose within your body. Proteins can be deaminated (remove the amino radical -usually by hydrolysis- from an amino compound) and then the carbohydrate portion again converts to glucose. Actually, your body will initially use the carbohydrates in your diet as a source of glucose for its glycolysis to pyruvate (convert to lactate under anaerobic conditions or broken down to water and carbon dioxide in the presence of oxygen), then the fatty tissue in your body, then the proteins will be deaminated so your body can get to the carbohydrate they contain. Were it not for what is referred to as the Krebs Cycle, your body could not use the glucose as described above to generate energy. The only option open to it would be anaerobic respiration or energy production in the absence of oxygen.

Food can have an effect on the brain. So, the brain can be excited by food. Therefore, excitotoxins are the amino acids with which we must familiarize ourselves. Amino acids are chemical building blocks that are used to create proteins. The body uses proteins for various functions. A notable function is that of anabolism whereby proteins are constructed within a cell. Proteins are always being broken down and must be replaced. This is the reason we look for a percentage of protein to be supplied in our food. However, some amino acids remain unaltered (are not made into proteins) for use by the brain.

Some amino acids are used as neurotransmitters. In addition, amino acids can be classified by their alkalinity and acidity. The classification is significant because it explains in which group an amino acid competes for absorption in the intestines and eventually the brain via the blood-brain barrier. Neutral amino acids fight for the same available position in the intestines. Thereafter, while in the bloodstream, the amino acids fight for a position in the brain. The competition of the amino acids can affect one's behavior.

Around the world, people are eating foods that will eventually cause them to react with erratic behavior, die from the ignorance of what it is referred to as food or a disease that the substance produces. As we eat and experience highs and lows, we fail to see that the body is struggling to remove poisons. We ingest partial foods and our bodies attempt to intelligently convert the substances into whole foods. However, this is carried out by the body robbing organs of nutrients. The body needs whole foods. If it does not receive them, it naturally converts the poisons and foodstuffs at a price that will eventually diminish energy levels and emerge as an illness. With the abundance of refined foods, heat altered foods, canned foods and frozen foods; we are guaranteed to encounter a chemical behavior modifier. Foods cause both physical and mental illnesses as it robs the body of nutrients.

Education is heavily marketed in countries that experience a sluggish economy. An over-abundance of degrees is encouraged for individuals that figure youth with degrees to be more wise and certainly, more economical for businesses that promote under-qualified personnel. The elderly are being misplaced and wisdom is being prematurely buried. And too, persons with the discipline and freedom to only pursue degrees as professional students believe that expensive information will make their life more promising and add value. And when degrees are not accessible, titles are more readily available;   sometimes, without an increase in pay. Yet, no field of medicine is scrutinized as much as the holistic health field. For this reason, the practitioner is forced to prove his or her skills or education. Nonetheless, education does not guarantee safety, the avoidance of death or great expectations for any client enduring pain or illness. Furthermore, education is no more the solution to poverty than hard work or communism. Yet, there is a formula to success and no one is sharing it despite what book sales project and over-paid lecturers swear. And to think that the only secret is that there are no secrets; lends credibility to privilege.

Wealthy associations, government and the media influence the visions of the populous. If a field can attain an endorsement from either genre, the people will appreciate it and purchase a service or product without hesitation because the people live by the notion that the government will not harm the people. Tons of funds are directed at marketing to push drugs that cannot heal opposed to educating the people to care for themselves because there is far less gains in freeing slaves. With every new food, new drug, new drink or alternative food, it becomes apparent that the primary concern for the manufacturer is profit. Just the idea of selling something backed by lies is empowering.

In the U.S., a chosen field of study is extremely important. Therefore, the school attended, title, level or years of education, and location of business are factored into how well a business or individual is perceived. And even the most unsuccessful person wants to identify with success in some form. For this reason, a many sick persons suffer for years before choosing an effective therapy that does not require one to be radiated or violated with chemicals. Undoubtedly, the most influential groups have manipulated the public's perception of holistic practitioners. This occurs anywhere that people are inspired to wear white because it is supposed to be the color of hope and the lab coat is the symbol of the healer.

The individual skill level is barely considered by the controlling associations that finance campaigns to discredit holistic health or practitioners that have not taken oaths to become licensed killers. Moreover, American chiropractors are addressed and treated as physicians. Whereas, in Mexico, the *quirofísico* and chiropractor - which are trained to use their hands more effectively than US chiropractors - are not readily viewed as doctors. Consequently, the American chiropractor is recognized and accepted by insurance companies as well. And we know that insurance is synonymous with money in any country. An American chiropractor with a table, a degree, a list of car accidents and a telephone can make a decent living without ever knowing the difference between the functions of muscles and the purpose of bones.

The true definition of doctor is derived from the Latin word *docere* which means to teach and one who has earned a doctorate degree. In essence, a true doctor is one who has earned a doctor of philosophy degree. Yet, the medical doctor is seen as the epitome of what a doctor should be; and thus, referred to as a 'real doctor'. Mind you, non-communicable diseases currently cause nearly two thirds of all deaths worldwide. However, the global concern about the increase of deaths from heart and lung disease, cancer and diabetes prompted the United Nations to hold a high-level meeting on non-communicable diseases in New York in September 2011 according to the World Health Statistics of mid-2012. Meanwhile, the people enthusiastically depend on men in white to cure and save them. The Telegraph newspaper of the United Kingdom reported in January 2013 that 43 hospital patients starved to death in 2012 and approximately 111 died of thirst. To no surprise, the Office for National Statistics reported that 287 patients were recorded, by physicians, to have been malnourished at the time of death. Another 558 had died in a state of severe dehydration. Consequently, people are dying in parts of the world considered to be far more advanced and civilized and still, the focus is on so-called dangerous herbs and natural, less toxic approaches to healing.

In Mexico, the naturopathic doctor is respected and recognized as a physician. However, in the U.S. the naturopath has to carry himself in a stiff, clinical, allopathic manner or be recognized as a phenomenon in order for the people to exalt and trust him or her. With notoriety, the skills, accomplishments or commitment of the practitioner is overlooked and their word becomes more presumptive. Unfortunately, this attitude will eventually sterilize and dilute the use of and application of botanicals.

Basic Principles of Natural Medicine

A number of holistic health practitioners that offer iridology, herbology, reflexology, massage or nutritional counseling are referred to as "doctor". Not all have been formally educated or trained. And for a percentage of practitioners, education will not, has not and cannot make a difference. Mexico has some of the most gifted yerberos, sobadores, curanderos, homeopatas, hueseros, parteras and quirofisicos that learned by participating and listening. Their expertise challenges the definition of ´formal education´. Regardless, there are principles that should be observed by persons wishing to heal or assist persons experiencing less than optimal energy levels.

Recognize the Healing Power of Nature	The practitioner should recognize that the human body has an innate capacity to heal and therefore, have the ability to instruct client in healing.
Locate and Eliminate the Cause	Find the cause of the disease or discomfort and eliminate it so that healing can occur. Assist client in reevaluating their lifestyle in order to identify the cause of disease and take corrective action.

Teach Health	Unlike the disease industry, teach clients how to achieve and maintain proper health. Ascertain that the client wants to participate in their healing.
Honor the Total Person	Recognize the whole person. The aspects of physical, mental and spiritual should be analyzed when educating a person in healing. The body should not be fragmented.
Prevent Discomfort or Dis-ease	Teach client how to achieve balance without introducing toxins.

The holistic health practitioner must be aware of the following information and avoid practices that infringe upon practicing medicine without a license. Of course, a number of modalities, herbal formulas and advice are imparted because the damage that occurs does not usually happen immediately.

Do No Harm	Natural practitioners should not use harmful substances, questionable herbal concoctions or ineffective alternatives.
Do Not Diagnose Disease	Practitioners can perform evaluations and analyses. However, the practitioner should avoid diagnosing the person.
Do Not Treat Disease	The practitioner teaches the client how to change the internal and external environment, but does not treat symptoms or a specific

	disease.
Do Not Prescribe Pharmaceuticals	Practitioner teaches the client how to make choices about their health while implementing fresh foods, herbal formulas, nutritional supplementation and natural modalities.

The socialized disease system of the U.S. is a safe haven for those making exorbitant salaries and those fortunate enough to get the treatments they need. Besides, the costs of healthcare and insurance coverage in America are unaffordable for an overwhelming number of Americans. Around 50 million people are uninsured, despite having employment. So, while some well-insured, privileged people may be over-medicated, poisoned and radiated, others are struggling for the simplest care. Of course, Mexico's acceptance of ethnomedicine is facilitated by the people's respect for the ways of their Ancestors and the practitioner's continuance of an established indigenous medical system. However, persons wishing to trust modern medicine, in an attempt to appear developed, are eligible for subsidized healthcare despite employment status. And with Mexico's large population, there are more than 3,000 private hospitals that offer care based on giving the individual the level of care that they can afford. And though, some of these hospitals have no nurses, laboratories or radiography equipment, they are able to do harm as a proto-type with nutrient-poor foods, toxic medications and service that is modeled after and branded by the disease industry. As Mexico changes from the ways of the old into a more developed country, it habitually adopts eurocentric methods that will prove to be more than innocuous.

We have been told that we can eat anything that we wish; as long as we pray, thank God and blindly trust the notion that the government would not approve of any foods or drugs that could do us harm. And of course, most of us believe that God would not create anything that would hurt us. However, we forget that the creation of God and creator of gods is motivated by control. Man will do harm because man can do harm. This fact becomes apparent with sickness and age. After ingesting toxins in the form of government approved medications, we eventually learn that the best weapon that we have against disease and rapid aging is the routine consumption of uncorrupted, fresh foods.

In Mexico, like any other place in the world, people are influenced by print ads, commercials, and what celebrities do on the big screen. Those whom are less fortunate do not avoid eating nutrient-poor, processed foods because they are not familiar with health and diet; but they choose to eat "anything" because they do not understand how what they eat will affect their health. Moreover, education is not a guarantee that people will do any differently or any better because the majority is taught that protein in the form of meat is necessary to prevent malnutrition. Certainly, finances or the pursuit thereof, play a role in what is chosen as a meal. This is more evident for persons that labor daily for 12 hours to earn 50 pesos, after spending up to eight pesos to arrive at their job, another 12 pesos for breakfast and 14 pesos for lunch. After totaling the expenditures for a work week of six days, very little money remains. This is the reason why a kilogram of eggs, a kilogram of tortillas, a kilogram of beans, a whole chicken and a portion of beef or pork are mandatory items on the grocery lists of most homes. And sadly, this forced habit creates a problem due to the lack of variety in terms of nutrients and of course, the consumption of flesh without fresh vegetables.

The power of government, whether socialist or democratic, pales in comparison to the groups that influence the psyche and habits of the masses. These same groups eventually influence governments. With every advertisement that we see, our creativity is dulled. The minds of men (that we never hear of or see) work hard to ascertain that we eat the foods that are less than nutritious; wear clothing and adornments that question our sexuality; and accept environmental toxins in the presentation of water, dental hygiene, medications and foodstuffs.

The mental processes of the masses are hardwired to deny that manipulation is in progress. Furthermore, education and money do not equip an individual with the necessary psychic self-defense needed to avoid being manipulated. And the idea of holding on to old traditions does little to deter the intentions of individuals whom consciously offer direction to any and every event.

The wires attached to our minds are being gently pulled as we move in a fashion that was designed by individuals that understood very little about ethnicity, culture or tradition before employing persons willing to commit treasonous acts such as betrayal. Regardless of where you live on the planet, you are eventually a participant in the democratic game of insanity that pushes consumerism. Of course, with the acceptance of American values and modernity, the Mexican populous will be subjected to mind molding, destruction of creativity and having their destinies planned before their conception.

In terms of propaganda, the holistic health field should never embrace the White Coat Ceremony or the white coat tradition. Today, only one in eight doctors wear white because Americans have learned that some patients are frightened by the traditional garb. And then there are people who do not trust doctors. Another reason for abandoning the white is due to the fact that the assumed visual symbol of hierarchy interferes with the progress of patient care and studies show that during a doctor's visit a percentage of patients experience "white coat hypertension" which causes their blood pressure to increase. Inharmoniously, a larger number of patients prefer the white coat because it separates the physician from the staff. Nevertheless, the disease industry has a record of problems that the holistic health industry cannot compete with.

Truth be told, possessions such as the white coat, watches, ties, rings and long sleeves should be banned for reasons of patient safety concerns. This act is equivalent to a fast-food employee sweating while running to work, through rush hour traffic and cooking or serving in the same clothing once their shift begins. In Canada, there are an estimated 220,000 hospital-acquired infections annually and as many as 12,000 deaths as a result. No one wants to know the truth about hospitals and doctors. Sure, medical doctors swear to do no harm, but as a professional courtesy they overlook the mistakes of their colleagues. The medical doctor is revered. So, natural physicians do not bother to challenge the errors of allopathic physicians either. This may be due to the comparison of educations and the misplaced competitiveness that exists amongst homeopathic and naturopathic physicians for one another.

In the U.S., surgeons operate on the wrong body part an average of 40 times per week according the Wall Street Journal. 1 in 4 persons that enter a hospital will be harmed by a medical error. The errors cost the disease industry tens of billions of dollars a year. Almost 30 percent of procedures, tests and medications are unnecessary. This percentage has to be flawed because persons being misdiagnosed and then prescribed medications are probably not factored into this equation. The mistakes do not deter people from trusting doctors because the waiting rooms and emergency rooms are always occupied. A doctor is automatically issued with charisma and trust because he, as a stranger, is capable of getting us to disrobe. He is not looking to diagnose holistically. Therefore, he is not looking for colors, feeling for vibrations or heat. He is clueless. He is far from being a conversationalist. He is barely studying the individual. And you will likely be misdiagnosed. If you do not complain, he is considered successful. If you do not die, he continues with the same, outdated, primitive methods of prescribe, cut and destroy.

The depressing number of medical care mistakes can also be attributed to the lack of hand-washing, but the real culprit is the cuff of the bacteria-laced white coat. While thinking and refusing to be wrong, most doctors fold their arms or put their hands in their pockets. In actuality, medical staff should shower and change clothing any time they leave the hospital or office. And lab coats shouldn't be treated as fashion wear. It is not my intention to dull the aura of godliness that comes with the white coat, but rather to demonstrate that the persons in the white coats are not without error. More importantly, people should know that the healthcare and medical industry is nothing more than a disease industry. It is easy for a person to think that they are sick, but it is guaranteed that a doctor knows exactly what is wrong. It doesn't matter if your ability to verbalize your pains and concern is subpar, medical doctors are capable of understanding what the patient needs. It is likely that the individual will leave the doctor's office or hospital with medication to start, a prescription for duration of contents, and a bill that does damage to one's budget and stress level. More importantly, a diagnosis for daily conversations will accompany most visitors because complaining about one's poor health is acceptable material for most conversations. Medical doctors are gods in the absence of pharmaceutical salesmen and whores in their presence.

Even the least educated citizen may suspect that TV commercials and news articles are not telling us the whole story. For the very few who take time to research beneath the surface of the daily programming, advertisements and social opinion and of course, who are still capable of independent thought, a somewhat darker picture begins to surface. The public will not always accept everything that the government says because everyone will not believe things such as HIV causes AIDS; the purpose of the health care industry is health; Americans have the best health in the world; insulin injections cure diabetes; vaccines prevent infectious diseases; pharmaceuticals restore health; you never outgrow your need for milk; no child can get into school without being vaccinated; the FDA thoroughly tests any and all drugs before they are available for use; fluoride protects the teeth; chronic pain is a natural consequence of aging; and/or aspirin prevents heart attacks.

No lie is insignificant. A lie is a lie! To paint a lie as white does not condone the intended purpose despite the lack of damage or results. Every government conditions its citizens not to question authority. However, this is your life! And in an effort to do the right thing, it is possible that one's choices of foods are not healthy and too, said selections are assisting the company that you wish to avoid to finance other dangerous products. Today, it is normal for Big Food corporations to invest in multiple brands and have the brands compete with one another. As a third of Americans are obese and childhood obesity is rising, the best approach is to not trust packaged foods or foods that last more than usual without refrigeration. The secret to health is really more about common sense than moderation. The body must expel any toxins that are ingested, inhaled or absorbed into the body. So, the idea of eating small amounts of poison and not expecting them to accumulate and cause harm is not normal even if it is common.

Ch 8 Medical Racism

The ethnomedical perspective of medicine has to consider melanin. And though, melanin is downplayed by the medical establishment as nothing more than pigmentation, it is intensely studied by scientists. Of course, they apply their theories to the science and confuse the populous into thinking that their practices are scientific.

Ethnomedicine has to recognize melanin and its importance or ignore African wisdom while committing ancestral treason because science is spiritual. To accept scientific myths and theories is an act of accepting compartmentalized concepts and half-truths based on European standards and comprehension. Moreover, ethnomedicine distinguishes between illness and disease by seeing disease as a biomedical condition and illness as a socio-cultural category.

Interestingly, ethnomedicine has the duty of acknowledging chlorophyll and its numerous wonders. Chlorophyll is empowered with the ability to regenerate our bodies at the molecular and cellular level. Furthermore, it cleanses the body, heals wounds, promotes the health of the digestive, immune, circulatory and detoxification systems and fights infection. The idea of not emphasizing what would be the melanin of plants and ignoring the role of melanin is another indication that medical science is practicing scientific racism by pushing pseudoscientific techniques and hypotheses to justify focusing on the privileged and overlooking the less fortunate. In actuality, medicine would be a legitimate science if it used data of melanin opposed to thinking that melanin is publicly equated with blackness and/or insinuates racial superiority.

"In humans, tyrosine, an amino acid, is the main nutrient. Tyrosine is a precursor of melanin and lays the foundation for melanin to be produced. They must contain an enzyme known as tyrosinase and copper to be able to use tyrosine to create melanin. In humans, there are three types of melanin. The first being Eumelanin which has a high electric charge, high molecular weight and density and gives rise to colors from dark brown to blue black.

A less dense form of melanin with lower molecular weight is known as pheo-melanin. It is also true that people with pheo-melanin have also quite a few more cancerous developments than those with Eumelanin."

Unblind Africanus of ***Blackherbals*.com**

Who Said You Were Sick?

Dr. Llaila Afrika has often stated that when a melanin dominant person is diagnosed as "sick", they are actually twice as sick. To explain, it is imperative that we understand that humans are grouped into   categories based on melanin content. The suspension of ethnicity or race is not possible in this explanation. The reader may assume that the author is racist for addressing this issue, but I am not. Mind you, I am of African descent. Therefore, I am Afrikan and unable to be "racist". However, I have learned to react to racism and at times, I make attempts to correct or change the conditions intended or created by racism. Lastly, I have received a more than adequate education in "white studies" and know that racism breathes and thrives when one race, class or group (not nationality) holds a disproportionate share of wealth, influence and power over other races, groups or nations and uses said wealth, influence and power to control, exploit, marginalize, exclude or lower in rank the targeted or despised group, nation or race. Oppressed peoples lack the financial or military resources to oppress or exhibit racism and are therefore, disqualified as racists. Nevertheless, for individuals that are recognizing, living, breathing and eating ethnomedicine, it is impossible to embrace, admire, imitate and push allopathic concepts without abandoning or dismantling the concepts established by Nature and African wisdom. Hippocrates is not the father of medicine and Greece is not the cradle of civilization.

The classifications of melanin in the body and skin are as follows:

TYPE	COLOR	RACE
6	Black, Blue-Black (MelaninDominant)	Africans (Afrakans, New Afrikans)
5	Black-Brown, Brown	Native Indians (Aztecs, Mayans, Incans etc.)
4	Brown, Red	Native Americans, Japanese
3,2	Yellow, Mixed, Mixed Brown	Orientals
1	White (Melanin Recessive)	Caucasians

Regardless of where you live, if your government has received any type of aid from the International Monetary Fund, housed the Red Cross, protected missionaries or allocated land for military bases, or accepted aid during an emergency, you have likely been exposed to the health standards of the European. Be it, baby formulas, daily recommended allowances of vitamins, disease reactions or anything to do with science, the information is based on the melanin content of melanin recessive beings. In addition, the majority of animals that are mistreated in medical laboratories are melanin recessive. The norm values of each race are different because biochemically speaking, each race is different. So, when a melanin dominant person is sick, they are being tested on the laboratory standards of a melanin recessive entity. And because the melanin dominant person does not meet the white standard, the person is not only sick – this person is twice as sick. Mathematically speaking, the melanin dominant person that is sick is beyond two times the standard.

The simplest way of measuring the response of melanin is by monitoring the pH and blood pressure. The potential of Hydrogen is an electrical measurement of urine and saliva. The urine exhibits the sympathetic activity of the Autonomic Nervous System and the saliva exhibits the nerve actions and reactions of the parasympathetic system. We must understand that this measurement does not determine the amount of pigmentation an individual has. Melanin can fluctuate and become deficient due to environmental exposure or the ingestion of toxins. Consequently, the body's need for melanin can be greater than the availability of melanin needed to fight disease. For this reason, an emphasis is placed on the use of herbs, essential oils, whole foods and the cancellation of processed foods.

A deficiency of melanin is apparent when the pH of urine is not a pH of 6.4 and the systolic pressure is above or below 120. The systolic pressure and the urine pH are related to the serotonin of the melanin. This is the male principle and recognizes acidity, the sympathetic nervous system, the left hemisphere of the brain, and the use of carbohydrates for energy.

In terms of the saliva, if the pH is not 6.4, there is a melanin insufficiency. And too, when the diastolic pressure of the blood is above or below the range of 80 there are melanin issues. The diastolic pressure and the urine are of the female principle and are related to the melatonin of the melanin and refer to the alkalinity, the usage of raw fats, parasympathetic nervous system, and the right hemisphere of the brain. It is possible to have a sufficient amount of melanin and the body may not be able to function properly or utilize the melanin. This may occur when the neurological and metabolic aspects of the body malfunctions due to a debilitated organ or system. Hormonal and gland problems can damage systems and compromise the ability of the body to use melanin, too.

It appears that disease industry is doing so much good, but a larger than necessary percentage of people die each year in hospitals, doctor's offices, at home or en route to home due to mistakes made my scientists, pharmaceutical companies, government agencies and doctors that refuse to acknowledge their oath. Medical racism is apparent even if it is not as obvious as iatrogenisis. A coin toss can get you disease or death because mankind is at odds with Nature. The melanin dominant being is functioning on a different frequency than melanin recessive beings. In simpler terms, melanin dominant people are gifted with ways to use melanin and undoubtedly their mind, body and spirit without fragmentation or denial of the existence of this particular trinity. Melanin is inside and outside of the body. Scientific myths do not want to share the genius of melanin because it is a civilizing chemical that reproduces itself, transforms in the blood, concentrates brain and nerve information and protects against free radicals. The Pineal Gland or what some refer to as the "third eye" secretes melanin. So, when the body is sick it is due to the mismanagement and neglect of the temple and the inability to see and sense based on the blindness of the third eye caused by immune suppressors such as foodstuffs, medications or recreational drugs. Neither living nor dying should be as expensive as marketing pimps have made it.

Marketers know that people trust packaging. As soon as the words natural, organic or pure are read, the product is automatically trusted. Consequently, there is a minute percentage of real food that can be found in stores that sell food. The stuff found in glass bottles, plastic bottles, cardboard boxes, plastic boxes, Styrofoam boxes, plastic bags, or frozen and packaged are preserved in some form after being killed or concocted. In addition, the word health is derived from an Old English word that meant wholeness, being whole, sound or well. If this definition holds true to theory, it would be safe to assume that a whole being needs whole foods, if they are to remain sound and well. Yet, we are duped into accepting words socially and of course, culturally. So, we rarely investigate what we say, think or believe. This is the reason that most people, when encountering or speaking of a vegetarian, assume that vegetarians only eat vegetables. The root of vegetarian is *vegetus* and it means "full of life" opposed to vegetable. Ironically, most vegetarians eat over-cooked vegetables or very few vegetables, at all. No one is safe! Health food stores employ dizzy, clueless persons to operate stores that carry items that are one or two ingredients less toxic than what the majority of the population is accustomed to buying in the Big Food chains. And the people that frequent such stores and restaurants pretend to have superior intelligence, while in all actuality, most harbor a cancerous, artificial intellect. With such toxic clerks, you are lucky to get the correct change in such stores.

Around the world, governments are practicing discriminatory and disproportionate laws by banning the sale of selected herbal medicinal products by individuals that are not registered as holistic practitioners. Licenses and permits (of any sort) never prove competence or knowledge. However, the licenses prove that the government has a voice in the direction of the licensed individual. The use of medicinal plants is the most common form of traditional medication worldwide because many people cannot afford the over-priced chemicals that are approved and sold as safe pharmaceuticals. The big corporations that fear a decrease in drug sales, lobby and pay for the government for regulation of herbal medicines under the premise that it is a key means of ensuring safety, efficacy and quality of herbal medicinal products.

Mexico has more than 5,000 medicinal herbs that have been explored by holistic practitioners, shamans and lay persons. Throughout the markets of Mexico, it is common to find herbs. And the memory (not to be confused with knowledge) of persons selling herbs is phenomenal. However, the government and big corporations have used their influence to make people question herbs, the salesperson, the holistic practitioner, the medical capabilities of herbs and whether or not they are safe. Yet, soil that has been saturated with pesticides, herbicides and any other poison that man has had to dispose of is trusted to provide nourishing foods for the people. Today, it is difficult for the foods to be one's medicine. And those that trust the medicines approved by the government eventually learn that the medications come with a number of problems. Some people call the problems side-effects. Yet, Nature's intentions are right and exact.

It must be agreed upon that all natural products are not edible, curative or safe. Again, just because a product receives government approval as a food or medicine does not mean that it is trustworthy or even a food. We assume that the ability to chew and swallow a substance makes it edible. However, there is no guarantee that the body will receive any nourishment, from any substance, packaged and sanctioned by any government.

The government is composed of people that, at one time, understood life, struggle, freedom, opportunity, change, and the pursuit of happiness. Somehow, people trust people that have lost their vision and compassion due to being desensitized by the smell of money and sense of power. The very people that control the gardens and hire people to prepare their meals are enjoying meals and learning to turn their heads at the notion that people are starving and dying from diseases caused by nutrient-poor soil, toxic drugs and the suspension of creativity or the pursuit of happiness. No one should assume that the government has the best interest of the people at heart because privilege and greed usually trumps generosity, promises and the needs of the people.

As people strive to become in-tune with nature and change poor habits that are promoted by marketers, the idea of growing herbs and foods in buckets or available space is becoming more prevalent. For this reason, no government should expect their employers - the people - to patent herbs that are not accompanied by millions of dollars or the outright intentions of earning money.

In Mexico, herbs are seemingly in abundance. Whether you want herbs in capsules, teas, or natural form - they are available. The government should have no part in this game, but the players should definitely rotate the herbs periodically, improve their knowledge of medicinal properties of herbs, stop undermining nature and speak up for their rights. The people should never give the government the right to control or sanction what Nature has freely offered as a gift to sustain life.

As organizations and governments gain control of the use of herbal medicinals, the number of deaths due to the body's inability to heal from toxins will increase. Some herbs contain toxins and still, the uninhibited existence of herbs is necessary while government intervention is not. However, herbs, such as those found in China, with high levels of arsenic and lead should be avoided. Moreover, people should reexamine their perception of steamed white rice and vegetables soaked in monosodium glutamate. Health products should be scrutinized like any product that one intends to ingest or apply to their skin.

Truthfully, herbs do not heal. As a matter of fact, we use herbs in an isolated manner that causes the herb to be recognized as a drug by the body. Those of us in tune with more urban vocabulary and politically correct terminology are so focused on planted-based dieting that we do not see herbs as plant-derived drugs. Again, the soil is an issue whether it yields pretty produce or not.

Learning to live properly opposed to living strong is in order. Replacing synthetic supplements with the practice of herbal supplementation is just as dangerous as using any toxin. Herbs can kill. Fortunately, most users lack the knowledge to use herbs in a harmful manner and the record of herbs is far better than that of medications, doctors and hospitals. A percentage of persons using herbal medicine never share with their physicians that they are using plant-derived drugs. Of course, the doctor compounds the problem by prescribing synthetic drugs to be coupled with the patient's ignorance and silence.

Surely, it is confusing to differentiate between what Nature offers and what man says. After all, genetically modified foods grow in the soil because scientists with knowledge of genetic engineering took the toxin-producing gene from the bacteria and introduced it into crops such as soy, papaya, corn, wheat, alfalfa, tomatoes, sugar cane, cantaloupe and sugar beets. Yes, roughly 94 percent of soy in the U.S. is genetically modified and used in soy products. There is no need to trust the opinions of persons addicted to foods that remind them of animal cookies and taste like rotting flesh. As of matter of fact, the people do not have to wait for research to be published that states how the human body can be genetically altered by poisons intended to destroy insects that were making us aware of the existence of poor quality produce. Again, Nature has her methods and man has intentions that appear to be god-like for only short periods of time.

Ch 10 Nature's Revenge

It is baffling to hear people talk about animal rights and/or animal cruelty while eating flesh and blood. And yet, animal cruelty occurs anytime that the industrial complex known as factory farming is involved. Factory farms continue to cram more animals into small spaces and separate animals from the natural order of living prior to initiating the ruthless process of preparing an animal to be slaughtered. In addition, circuses are not any better. I love the *UniverSoul Circus* because it is fun, soulful and entertaining. People of color from around the world display feats of courage and strength that selectively include camels, dogs, horses, elephants, and tigers. Until the early part of 2012, while visiting Jacksonville, Florida, I had never given thought to circuses as being cruel. Granted, the smell was always horrible and I was never hungry because of it. The smell of feces, of any type, always altered my appetite. Yet, I saw no wrong in the captivity of animals destined to entertain or attack. However, the protestors with large images of animals chained, caged, whipped and adorned in silly costumes left an indelible impression on my psyche. I had always enjoyed seeing the show under the "big top" in Atlanta, but that particular night in Florida somehow changed my outlook of different earthlings being used for the purpose of entertainment and the testing of chemicals.

My avoidance of flesh and blood is not political. I am not the type of person that crashes a vehicle to avoid an animal crossing the interstate. I will not attempt to liberate animals in captivity and risk being bitten in the process and/or arrested. In addition, I am not impressed with trend diets, marketing-inspired terms or methods that promise everything while delivering nothing.

Obviously, there is no sane method for getting any creature mentally ready to be butchered or held in captivity. Not even war in the name of religion or allegiance to one's country can do that. Man has learned to use parts of animals that go beyond flesh and bone. One may think that man is resourceful, but his actions have proven to be nothing more than conniving as he uses what he can and disposes of other things by finding ways to hide them in products that we eat or drink. Science uses various names to conceal the truth. Long after we are exposed to the dangers of scientific practices and names, we learn the nasty truth. To a degree, everyone is subjected to animal products. Of course, vegetarians have learned to use replacements to obtain their desire for meat. But due to the trickery of science and marketing, they have not fully abandoned meat. Certainly, milk from goats and cows are mandatory for most people attempting to avoid the ingestion of flesh. However, cheese and eggs are favorite choices of the best and most misinformed vegetarians.

Marketing gurus have found ways to conceal animal products as rennet, emulsifiers, suet, whey, glycerin, tallow, capric acid, and stearic acid. We are eating enzymes from the stomach of calves in cheese, fatty acids in ice cream, animal fat in chocolate, lard in the pretty pastries, membranous tissue of cows in potato chips that we can't just eat one of, glycerin and lanolin in chewing gum and calcium stearate (tallow)in hard candy. We can't trust the labels on highly preserved foods. Anyone wishing to avoid meat must read or improve their memory. Caesar dressing and Worcestershire sauce contain anchovies; canned soups contain fish stocks, beef stocks and chicken stocks. Again, animals are so deep into our lives and psyche that most of us want foods that look like animals or taste like animals. Some beers, jellies, marshmallows, gummy bears, gelatins, jelly, refried beans and tortillas contain animal products as well. If we intend to decrease animal cruelty and diseases caused by our consumption of meat and animal products, we will have to do our due diligence in determining what is safe. The government is crawling with people that are intrigued by what they can do covertly. The powers that be are not fascinated with money because they realize that wealth is nothing without labor. People, for the most part, are necessary. Powerful people look to control the "have nots". Of course, the stomach is the easiest way to control the masses. Anyone who disagrees with the ease of control has evidently not learned how labor intensive growing food can be. And too, those whom are afraid of work cannot speak of true liberation or sovereignty.

Despite our views of vegetarianism or omnivorism, we are conditioned to accept *speciesism* in order to justify our abusive and inconsiderate slaughter and consumption of beings that do not communicate or carry on daily lives as humans. Speciesism permits us to make a disconnection between all life forms and nature. According to *Vegan.com*, speciesim is a failure, in attitude or practice, to accord any non-human being equal consideration and respect. This concept should not be surprising because enslavers justified enslaving Africans by defining "the original man and woman" as *subhuman*. To this very day, persons of African descent — to include those of denial about their origin - must deal with the residue of such toxicity. Again, the toxins affecting our lives are not just in the form of medications and marketing.

Many people think of animal cruelty as being limited to people mistreating their dogs or subjecting them to brutal fights for profit. However, Mexico City has an issue of stray dogs and cats. The exact number is unknown. Yet, estimates range from the hundreds of thousands to upwards of five million. How is this possible? A many of these pets were once gifts to someone in need of love or a lesson of responsibility. But as serious as the problem may be due to alleged mauling deaths by stray dogs, it is the least of the animal cruelty concerns. Animals do not write or speak. Therefore, the thought of animals being accused of participating in the unnecessary deaths of human lives is just as cruel as the senseless deaths that continue the legacy of untimely deaths. And then there is the use of animals for testing products that may be too dangerous for humans. The rule for product use must be simplified: If you cannot eat the product, do not trust the product on your skin.

The food industry is responsible for the most horrific animal cruelty because living beings are harvested to entertain the desires of people that see flesh and blood as mandatory items at any meal. The conditions under which these animals are briefly raised are extremely cruel. The idea of raising animals in confined areas that prevent muscle development, breaking the beaks of chickens and feeding diseased animal parts and inedible products to animals intended for human consumption is definitely cruel. Imagine the cattle that you are prepared to consume this week being branded, dehorned, chained to a bar, force-fed antibiotics and later transported in conditions that contribute to death. For the cattle that do not die, they will receive a rod in the brain and a thrust to their head. Still, they must be hoisted, cut and bled. Some of the cattle instinctively continue their fight and struggle to live amongst earthlings that see no harm in hurting species that are different or more melanin dominant. Death by disease or death by process - even the dead animals will mysteriously make it to market. Sure, it is cruelty for the animal, but it is even more unfair for the health of humans relying on animal flesh for their well-being.

The misinformation surrounding the definition of protein and its necessity has confused the larger percentage of people. Most of them cannot imagine a plant-based diet. So, the idea of discussing the required acreage for animals versus digestible protein is useless because feeding the world is not a priority. And as long as people demand animal flesh, they will get it without asking for changes in the factory farming industry practices. After all, mandating organic, free-range practices do not guarantee that consumers will get sane, healthy, chemical-free flesh that has not been tainted with the blood of dying, diseased animals or an abundance of fecal matter. Furthermore, the notion of conducting the killings of animals in a humane manner is inane. Murder is murder! And if the animals are to be slaughtered for the provisions of other beings, there really is no mentally stable way of doing it. It is a fact that the animals will suffer when killed by any means that does not use an expensive euthanasia solution. And eating less meat or avoiding meat will not stop the slaughter because other uses will be found for the animals. I reiterate, I do not advocate the idea of saving animals before saving one's self.

Natural Reactions?

The usual Saturday morning with a box of cereal and cartoons, laced with subliminal messages, have exposed most children to commercials geared at promoting bad foods and anti-social behavior. Parents, public education, and social conditioning have created an out-of-control child that can easily be compared to an ogre. This monster eats any and every thing, at any time of day. Before a meal can be removed from the system, more meals are eaten. This monster lives on the *pleasure principle*. No pill, no surgery and no diet can domesticate such a monster.

Mankind is wired to be both cruel and sensitive, evidently. Mankind destroys forest land for the construction of buildings that will eventually pollute streams and the air with industrial waste. Of course, mankind goes into countries to steal produce that offers nutrients that are unknown to most people and afterwards, they return to sell them to the same people in a form that is poisonous to the body. In addition, mankind destroys the natural eco-system while demolishing rainforests. This may appear to be an environmental issue, but it is indeed cruelty in terms of the human lives, plant life and animal life that depend on said ecosystems for life.

64

However, human behavior is contributing to the reduction of the human population through losses caused by natural disasters and infectious diseases. Nature does not discriminate and it never has to be kind. Moreover, man is no match for Nature; she does not need man in order to exist. Regardless, man will continue to challenge Nature, attempt to control Nature and even try to duplicate Nature. Man is only seeing things that are visible without considering the responsibilities of plants and microbial life forms that sustain human life.

As viruses and bacterium become more resistant to man-made drugs that line the shelves of pharmacies, man has to ponder the idea of returning to Nature sooner than later. Hopefully, this is accomplished before nature generalizes the actions of persons whom have no respect for life or nature and retaliates. It is obvious that we are not all the same. The presence of melanin (more than pigmentation) makes it clear that we are different. Nonetheless, we are all connected. The people, plants, animals and the planet must deal with the continuing effect of man's greed and decisions. Based on sound, right reasoning, man has a sacred obligation to obey the unwritten rules of nature. Whenever man breaks the laws, he violates his own "true nature" and automatically initiates a level of dis-ease that Nature never intended to enforce. This is not to say that nature is gentle because nature is indifferent. Yes, Nature is beautiful. Nature is indiscriminate; and habitually offers rewards and penalties. Nature is willing to survive at any cost. We will eventually learn that we cannot defeat Nature. And our attempts to fight Nature are nothing more than futile. It is imperative that we appreciate the ways of our Ancestors in our pursuit of modernity because man has become very arrogant and disrespectful. For this reason, if we are to use anything from any people, with ideologies that are foreign to those of our Ancestors, it must be from a perspective of our own culture. Besides, we will always be at the mercy of Nature and the grace of our Ancestors.

Ch 11 Dis-ease and Dependence

The thought of food combinations come to mind with ease; peanut butter and jelly, milk and cookies, meat and potatoes, steak and shrimp, cheese and crackers, and of course, bacon and eggs. Everybody has a favorite combination. And very few people understand the dangers of processed foods or the fact that food can be addictive. I regularly speak to people who claim they do not eat much. However, a percentage of them eat throughout the day and awake during the night to visit the refrigerator, if food isn't kept at bedside. And the most uneducated of the "rarely eat" category do not believe that they are eating because they never put their food on a plate or bother to sit at a table. Some people believe that every meal must include meat, bread and at least one over-cooked vegetable. Moreover, the aforesaid group of people has pot bellies and love handles. This is not coincidental or due to aging. However, disease and air are trapped in such toxic bodies.

The idea of being addicted to food is difficult for sick people to imagine despite the fact that they add seasoning to their food before tasting it, eat whether they are hungry or not, eat while sick, eat while watching television, snack between meals, think of food when they are not eating, eat while driving and plan their schedule with food in mind. The toxicity and acidity of the selected foods will be stored in the fat cells. Naturally, the fat cells will swell and cause the person to gain weight. By detoxifying and alkalizing the fat cells, we can release what has been stored and the person can lose the unnecessary weight. Fat is not healthy. And culture or the lack of income should not be an excuse to be unhealthy.

The result of most scientific research seems to do nothing more than add to the mountain of diet recommendations and nutritional theories that confuse the masses. The confusion is a clever method to promote consumerism and dis-ease as we pretend to choose the best of what is nothing less than malicious products. It is obvious that the research is only done to justify the receipt of grants and increase marketing. Clever marketing makes tap water in fancy bottles more attractive and cheap grains frosted with sugar in the form of breakfast cereals extremely profitable.

It is definitely time for a paradigm shift because the belief that three meals are necessary is a paradigm that is helping to kill the world much faster than bullets. No one is safe. There are diets advertised as being better than other diets. Yet, every diet implies a continued intake of food. We are enjoined to eat 5 to 8 small meals a day; increase intake of protein; eat a big breakfast; eat soups; drink gallons of lemon, honey, herb mixtures; eat loads of calcium; take supplements; take diet pills; eat whole wheat or count calories. However, be it cooked food or raw food, the body eventually requires rest and detoxification. Commercials and the disease industry have been instrumental in teaching us to enjoy life and eat, eat, eat. We pay more for junk food because we are convinced that we don't have time to prepare proper meals. Sadly, the foods of choice are not accompanied by happiness and each meal is not without risk. Consequently, no event is complete without something to eat.

It is indeed possible for an individual to improve their health, lose weight, and increase their metabolic rate. It is not as difficult as persons selling metabolic diet plans would like for us to believe. Metabolism refers to the processes that the body needs to function properly. Basal Metabolic Rate (BMR) is the amount of energy, expressed in calories, which a person needs to keep the body functioning while at rest. Such processes are breathing, blood circulation, cell growth, controlling body temperature, nerve function, brain function and muscle contractions. The basal metabolic rates affect the rate that a person burns calories and ultimately whether or not they maintain, gain, or lose weight. The basal metabolic rate accounts for about 60 to 75% of the calories that are burned each day.

Most people cannot go three hours without eating. However, they are still in a "fed state" - metabolically speaking, when they decide to ingest more food. The majority of over-eaters have not digested and assimilated the previous meal and yet, they want to add more food. Unfortunately, most of the chosen foods have toxins. How can the unprocessed food be referred to as energy when the person is tired after eating and still hungry with the same food still trapped in their body?

The misunderstanding of energy and so-called energy workers are confusing subjects. And many practitioners enter into the field of healing because they believe that they can heal. Actually, they are not healing anyone. Furthermore, if they do not understand energy, they likely will not understand the difference between a melanin cluster and how energy that is held in a location may be referred to as a blockage. It is beyond semantics and the need to earn a living has enabled sick people to oversee sickly people.

People are often confused about how they feel because various factors contribute to a feeling of vagueness or an ambiguous and non-specific condition. This is easily expressed as dis-ease or illness. Contrarily, abnormalities in an organ or system of the body are characterized as a disease because it is considered to be a diagnosable condition. Medical science is hardly a science. And yet, it serves a purpose that is rarely challenged and only beneficial in emergency situations. If we are sick, our immune system will fight the invasive organism to maintain health and prevent abnormalities. Once the immune system has successfully defeated the foreign invader, it creates antibodies to protect the body from getting the same illness in the future. As we encounter new diseases, our bodies thoughtlessly create more antibodies. It is possible for the body to be exposed to a number of foreign substances and never show any signs or symptoms. Regardless, our bodies will create antibodies to prevent any illness in the future. Ironically, with HIV, we have been informed that having antibodies is life-threatening. However, when a person has the antibodies, they don't really have the virus. However, this is the science that governs our life and the industry to which we have become dependent.

Ch 12 Combative Tactics

War is a true money maker and of course, it boosts the expectations of any group that may benefit. Wars get results; some good and some bad. If a country is not at war with another nation, it will find some home-grown group in its own country to wage war against. And if a government really wants to manipulate the people, it can wag the dog. Yes, governments can be creative, conniving, and sinister. Throughout the world, governments use the same tactics to manage, gain trust and regulate the meek.

Entertainment comes in a variety of forms. We are bombarded with false information, the lives of confused celebrities and of course, sports. The brain is constantly receiving thoughts and images. And once we think we have a break from the madness, the images reappear in our dreams. Sadly, a number of dreams are compounded by the intake of sugar and other substances that are ingested and assumed to be innocuous. The ability to differentiate fact from fiction is not easy for persons that have been subjected to superstition, religion, government, social dogma and too much TV. We live in a world where the truth is unbelievable and making the populous believe the truth is nearly impossible.

When the disease industry and scientific community are not employing combative measures to kill something such as a fictitious disease, they are certainly pushing fear on the populous. We are constantly told that we may catch a cold, catch a fever, catch the flu, catch a virus or even catch AIDS. Whether one is ready or not, athletic or not, or looking for recreation or not — the government is poised to sanction lies which are designed to wreck the creation of life, and suspend the notion of liberty and make the pursuit of happiness less appealing. In actuality, we are not catching anything. Whatever disease it is that we will be diagnosed and doomed to death with by self-confident physicians, whether right or wrong, is already within us and waiting to be activated. We contribute to the progress of the disease with the manner in which we think. This is not to say that we think ourselves into a state of illness, but that we have been taught how to react to disease based on how society defines it. However, we can think ourselves into sickness or display hypochondriacal behavior.

Pharmaceutical companies stay ready to scrimmage with anyone who dares to challenge them because the objective (money) is quickly accomplished and always available for military type endeavors that are as routine as a game of chess. Besides, good marketing, maniacal lawyers and one-eyed governments give Big Pharma the courage to do to the people as they desire. The employee of the people, the government, lacks courage or incentive to stand up to Big Pharma, Big Business, or anyone with financial stability or the option to do business elsewhere.

Disease is considered to be a loss of immunity in the disease business. In addition, disease is recognized as an immune system failure. However, the discomforts and illnesses that we routinely endure and label as disease are the body's attempt to maintain balance through a process of cleansing. In other words, if you do not detoxify your body, the body will do as it must in order to be pain-free, stress-free, and drug-free. The body is familiar with functioning properly even when the individual has learned to accept pain as a part of life. So, the appearance of warts, blisters, sores, acne, rashes, inflammations and the various drainages of mucus are proof that the body is aware of a problem and rightfully, cleaning the temple. The unsightly signs are normally labeled as "contagious". Such nonsense is actually a European superstition. However, it is imperative that we recognize the visual signs as indications that the intended methods of elimination are not working properly. The visual signs of cleansing are only dis-eases, but that which has caused the accumulation of waste can be viewed as the disease, if a disease or diagnosis is necessary. There really is no need to treat the dis-ease because the focus should be on the elimination of the dead cells and toxins.

It is more likely that a person diagnosed with a chronic disease will die from medication before dying from the disease they have been diagnosed to have. Bacteria are always present in the body. Bacteria, viruses and Nature are not anti-life. Nonetheless, melanin and the presence of bacterial flora in the digestive system dictate what an individual can or cannot eat. The bacterial flora also metabolizes the food, neutralize impurities and eliminate toxins.

By accepting bits and pieces of scientific ignorance, we are being damaged in bits and pieces that eventually show our ignorance with each pill that we swallow and assist with carbonated beverages. Convoluted talk about diseases such as AIDS or the popularized view of HIV causing AIDS has become somewhat taboo as the number of HIV cases, in the gay community, has doubled in the last 20 years according to new research. This has happened without the knowledge of the people or perhaps, the fear factor. However, the numbers do not indicate an epidemic.

AIDS and HIV have always served as more of a sociopolitical construct to promote fear and increase pharmaceutical sales than a disease. I recall being taught in school that AIDS could lie dormant in the body for 10 to 20 years. The suggestion was mind-boggling and yet, the information about AIDS always seemed to be different. AIDS was killing people; not as many as the government and media reported. They used estimates and mathematical formulas that made funeral directors study the deduction theorem and reexamine their marketing abilities. The nightly news carried stories of this sex organ disease every night: Crime and AIDS. We learned who had been arrested or who was thought to be armed, dangerous and on the run. And of course, we heard horrific stories of individuals who'd died of a disease that was so intelligent that it targeted particular activities and a particular group or ethnicity - naughty or nice. This was the climax of "penis envy" and melanin reduction. Regardless of the crime, governments do not blame themselves, police themselves, or arrest themselves when they can point the finger, cajole the people and if necessary, governments can unapologetically recuse themselves. The business of disease is corrupt. And what is so frightening is that a doctor has a license to kill a patient, but a government can kill an entire nation while the people wait patiently for the government to save them. No one is safe!

AIDS is seemingly a discriminatory disease, if it is even a disease. After all, it is said to be a syndrome because it is a group of diseases, clinical signs and symptoms that benefit hospitals, doctors, insurance companies and the manufacturer of the harmful drugs that eventually cause an individual to acquire an immune deficiency. AIDS has been referred to as being contagious. It has been called an epidemic. It has been everything that it appears not to be. It only wants certain kinds of people. But the idea of it finding a host, invading the host and waiting until it was or is ready to "attack" was stressful in the 80s and 90s and it has to be stressful, today. People that were not paid to study the virus relied on government circulars and the media to bring the truth. However, the news personalities are paid to be puppets; some people call them actors.

Before the digital age, watching the evening news was as sophisticated as reading the Black Enterprise, Wall Street Journal or the Robb Report. It was believed that the major networks would not lie to the people and the world was actually flat despite findings to prove otherwise. Besides, the more important viewers were supposedly too educated to accept mistruths. And a many of them were not being affected by the business of AIDS or the ruthlessness of the minds behind the AIDS conspiracy.

Imagine a glass of contaminated drinking water while vacationing in a third world country. Is the bacterium in the glass of water contagious? Is it more potent than what we have been taught about AIDS? Does it cause you to panic? Does contaminated water kill as many people as AIDS? Is there a pill or condom to prevent the dangers of contaminated water? Have the people been conditioned to fear contaminated water more than AIDS? That which is seen as the weaker or less harmful of the two problems – the contaminated water – is being eliminated shortly after the recipient has gargled or drank it. Let's say that it takes 2 to 4 hours for the water to have an effect. Your stomach bubbles and pressure builds in your body. After the initial elimination of the foreign substance, your body continues to make corrections. Surely, you can imagine this because you have experienced this so-called dis-ease. Yet, with AIDS you are supposed to believe that it is capable of sneaking into the body undetected and hiding without your body being alarmed, inquisitive or protective. Your cells just sit around doing nothing more than watching a stranger in the temple – for years. Influenzas have come and flown away, but none were as destructive and magical as this phenomenon that has bankrupted families, destroyed marriages, challenged Nature and questioned God. This is an example of bad science, bad parenting issues, bad tempers and certainly, a bad idea for making money: all are coming home to roost.

Surprisingly, water related diseases kill an estimated 3.4 million people each year. According to water.org, 780 million people lack access to clean water or an improved water source. Fecal matter is the cause of most illness. Only 10% of waste water receives treatment while the remainder is sent to available water sources. Sadly, more people have a cellular phone than toilet. Every 20 seconds a child dies from an illness that is water related. This fact, alone, does not give credence to the germ theory, but instead places spotlight on the issues of developing countries. As for AIDS or HIV, it is nothing in comparison to contaminated water and you don't need a foundation, flawed test for detection or a bunch of paid MDs and PhDs to determine the obvious.

It is reported that every 9.5 minutes, in the U.S., a person is infected with HIV. The study is not clear on whether the person is diagnosed with HIV or if the virus has been detected because there is no test to diagnose HIV. Actually, there is no test to detect HIV. The test is designed to detect HIV antibodies. Furthermore, the rise in HIV cases seems to be the clever marketing of drug companies which has misled the gay community. The new drugs have convinced users to believe that unsafe sex is permissible. Consequently, there is no proof that the use of condoms will make the participants of any type of sexual activity any safer. Regardless, it is believed that between 1990 and 2010 that more people engaged in sex without condoms. Supposedly, this led to a rate increase of 26% amongst homosexuals not using condoms and an increase of 76% of homosexuals being infected in the U.S. It is believed that the availability of antiretroviral drugs was the reason that a percentage of homosexuals refused to use condoms. After all the turmoil of the 80s and 90s and countless campaigns promoting the use of condoms, it is hard to believe the absence of condoms increased the number of HIV or that people would risk their health for a number of pleasurable moments that could result in agony and untimely death. Perhaps, numbers are being crunched to qualify institutions for grants. Few industries offer financial aid like that of AIDS or Cancer. And no industries can quite arrest logic like that of the disease industry, theme parks and marketing.

There is so much to be learned about disease, but understanding superstitions, military mode of thinking (not conspiracy theories) and lies is mandatory. Politicians cannot fix the problems because they are easily attracted to and absorbed by the problems. The explanation of disease and the theories accompanying disease have not made the populous any healthier. And in terms of AIDS or HIV, the CD4 cells (helper cells) are no longer considered a reliable marker to predict the progression of AIDS. And though, we have been told that a body that has been infiltrated by AIDS cannot fight off opportunistic diseases, this is a mistruth. The AIDS business is not any different than the cancer business; they both look for ineffective preventions to justify their continuous campaigning for money while stalling to find cures. Cures come with a limited potential for income, but the art of selling lies comes with a residual income.

Surprisingly, healthy people can have low CD4 counts as well. A count of 350 is common amongst people that are HIV-negative. However, a normal CD4 range is between 500 and 1500 cells in a cubic millimeter of blood. Still, the helper cell count can vary, at any time, in a 24 hour period. And if an individual is struggling with lack of sleep, a poor diet and stress, the person can be considered HIV-positive. Furthermore, the presence of HIV antibodies would normally indicate a past infection rather than a present one, if the person is not showing any signs of sickness. Look! A person can be diagnosed as having AIDS if they are HIV positive and have one of the thirty diseases associated with AIDS or they can have AIDS if they are HIV positive and have a CD4 cell count of less than 200. AIDS, the super-serious disease, requires other diseases to qualify it as a disease. AIDS is not an epidemic and it is not evolving as strongly as the plethora of European superstitions that attract billions of dollars. The AIDS industry has attracted enough money to afford a cure, but this has not happened because possibility of the disease is greater than the probability. Therefore, there is no cure because the discovery of cause is still questionable.

Ch 13 A Border South of the U.S.?

Every seven minutes a person dies of cancer in the country of Mexico. However, in the United States it is more common to read statistics that show the influx of immigrants coming through Mexico and into the land of opportunity than it is to read the number of companies migrating to Mexico to save money on labor costs in an effort to pocket money for persuading or dissuading the government. So, the idea of anyone knowing or caring about medical statistics in Mexico is unrealistic. Perhaps, the attention given to statistics in Mexico is not as germane as those of the United States. Nonetheless, diabetes, heart disease, cerebrovascular disease, cirrhosis of the liver and kidney failure are a few of the leading causes of death in America's backyard.

Mexico is ranked amongst the fattest countries in the world. And depending on the source, it is surprisingly ranked as the highest for childhood obesity. A quick, daily, common meal that lacks variety and an annual consumption of soft drinks that totals more than 14 billion dollars is not easy to scrutinize while en route to modernization. Yet, more than 38% of teenagers are overweight and gradually adding to the weight of Mexico's dilemma. And despite the amount of food eaten in this country, malnutrition is an issue that should concern every individual without the consent or attention of the government.

Of course, the repetitive presentation of numbers do very little to incite fear, induce trust or curve the ignorance of the populace. It may only be information that justifies the fact that disease and healthcare is only about business. People do not believe that harm can find them — until they are weak, hopeless and helpless. At this point, the smartest and strongest of individuals find themselves trusting egocentric, over-educated puppets that favor technology, recommend surgery, prefer pharmaceuticals and routinely decide a diagnosis, within 20 seconds, based on symptoms.

Ironically, throughout the world, the leading causes of death are heart disease, stroke/cerebrovascular disease, lower respiratory infections, chronic obstructive pulmonary disease, diarrheal diseases, HIV/AIDS, lung cancers, tuberculosis and diabetes. Undoubtedly, some problems are worse than others in Mexico and the United States. And the idea of naming diseases does not allow the sick to deal with their   problems any easier because misdiagnosis leads to the patient receiving medication for an illness that does not exist and too, the possibility of developing problems from the toxic medicaments which the body was not designed for. Undoubtedly, the act of naming symptoms only adds to the already increasing stress coupled with nutrient-poor foods, costly medications and the disintegration of family with modernity.

Ethnocentrists have gone through pure hell to educate the downtrodden, overlooked, abused and forgotten. Of course, their efforts pale in comparison to the well-dressed lobbyists with quick tongues and endless funds to woo, bribe and misinform the biggest threat to the God-given right of freedom. Yes, Big Business is serious about business! And though, the common masses are told to fight for their country in order to prove that they love it, the country (despite location) fails to love the people. Moreover, those whom are chosen or elected to uphold the constitution, defend said nation, and represent the people quickly become puppets of the elite and swear to oaths that permit them to forget what they have promised the common people. Therefore, healthcare is amongst the greater needs and concerns of those that are heavily taxed and too, those that can only pray for relief. Of course, it is not needed in the form of The Patient Protection and Affordable Care Act (*Obamacare*) because it cannot be over-emphasized that some things don't work in any country or on any day.

Today, the internet is inundated with articles on health and new-age solutions offering antiquated jargon - with an updated twist of confusion - and promises to teach one how to heal their bodies with the purchase of a gadget, a therapeutic touch coupled with hot oil, hot stones or a non-holistic therapist enduring more dis-ease than the client. Surely, the majority of persons have experienced a special diet amongst the pyramids of synthetic foods and poor combinations. Some information suggests that nutrient-starved persons consume a diet composed of super-nutrients or more food than the body should attempt to digest in order to get the necessary nutrients. Undoubtedly, if pain accompanies the person, they will easily swallow more herbs and/or synthetic concoctions than nature produces. Eventually, the manipulative guru-types convince the sick that a change of heart will cure their ills after a disgruntled, unemployed individual with useless degrees becomes a life coach because they failed in their previous field of study and have been employed to reprogram the thoughts of sick people. In addition, a percentage of the persons that make purchases of life-altering information rarely study or apply the information. A number of these individuals find themselves in the hospital or using borrowed prescriptions when over-the-counter medications fail.

Everyone is capable of healing with the life force that operates under the direction of the subconscious mind. However, the secret lies in the comprehension of the life force and its ability to release tension while stimulating cells to vibrate in harmony. Certainly, we all have to learn to look within ourselves with the use of visualization, prayer and meditation. There is nothing magical or impossible about healing or the capabilities of the human body. Sure, we are over-worked, busy, tired, lazy and willing to wait until age slows us down or dis-ease humbles us. But we really have no excuses for succumbing to disease, if we are living as we were designed. It is not difficult for us to move in the direction of healing without the use of toxic medicaments that do nothing more than mask pain. And despite the numerous books that speak of healing, the language is often too difficult to understand or it is simply beyond the capabilities of the author that writes as a gifted healer.

The subject of expiration is definitely worth meditation because even babies die. There is no adequate amount of words to philosophize the abbreviation of life without the realization of struggles or joys of living. Of course, some struggles can be avoided. Regardless of one's philosophy, everything that vibrates has a lifespan. Our desires and fears prevent us from letting Nature take her course. Despite our disobedience, struggle or inability to properly survive, we always want more life, more time or another chance. Once Nature has decided that something is no longer needed, the timing devices of chromosomes, called telomeres, continue the process of natural order. At this point, the things that we have relied upon such as money, higher learning, religion, God, technology, pharmaceuticals, cosmetics, surgery and science become ineffective and undoubtedly, obsolete.

The subject of drugs cannot be addressed without the understanding of what a drug really is. Money, sanitary practices, packaging and persuasive marketing do not determine whether or not a drug is safe, natural or effective. And an endorsement by a medical doctor definitely does not ascertain that the drug will not do harm. Furthermore, purchasing a product from a health food store does not mean that you will avoid poisons.

Drugs can be made from inorganic or organic matter. Nonetheless, the body immediately recognizes synthetic chemicals as the biochemistry changes with the introduction. Of course, drug is defined as a substance that has a physiological effect when ingested or otherwise introduced into the body, in particular. However, it should be noted that any substance derived through a process in which a substance is made of a concentration taken from an isolated substance is a drug. Vitamins, minerals and amino acids, among other things, are drug concentrates that are used to treat dis-ease, as well. Any isolated, concentrated substance can cause nutritional and chemical imbalances.

The fact that the body is viewed as a machine gives meaning as to why the manufacturers of drugs react inhumanely. Once the body is attacked by a disease, a drug is used to attack the disease. Unfortunately, the drug attacks the body as well. The disease industry treats disease as a poison. Therefore, stronger poisons are used to attack the assumed poison.

The use of the word natural makes it difficult for the majority to understand that food and herbs are drugs when the state is changed and at times - in their natural state. Once the herb or food is heated, the nutrients are concentrated and the medicinal properties are extracted. Thus, the state of the herb or food has changed and should be recognized as a drug.

Drugs interact with receptors on cells and enzymes in the cells. Drugs can be allopathic, homeopathic or naturopathic; and most drugs are poisonous. With the use of allopathic drugs, a second illness is produced. This particular illness excites a biochemical, immune reaction that supposedly rids the body of the created illness and possibly the initial illness. Such shallow thinking is the reason that few people are healed or cured. They simply experience a suspension of pain or a disappearance of symptoms. In terms of homeopathic drugs, the illness is replicated and introduced in a percentage that is expected to cause the body to react and attack the illness that it was initially unable to detect and destroy. And the natural approach is still a drug. However, it is not considered toxic. Regardless of the presentation of said herb, the immunity of the body is nourished and strengthened.

Again, removing substances from the natural state is the act of creating a drug. For example, the idea of sweeteners being derived from agave, maple, corn, beets, sugar cane, barley, rice, coconut or stevia and isolating it into a concentrate is altering the natural state and therefore, making a drug. The same can be said of polished white rice, oil, and white flour. Oil should be naturally obtained from plant foods opposed to being extracted and concocted for purposes of liquid, margarine or butter. We ingest partial foods and our bodies attempt to intelligently convert the substances into whole foods. However, this is carried out by the body robbing organs of nutrients. The body needs whole foods. If it does not receive them, it naturally converts the poisons and foodstuffs at a price that will eventually diminish energy levels that emerge as an illness.

Ironically, we habitually become more addicted to the presence of food, taste of food and the act of pretending to chew with each meal that we eat. This is due to the unnatural modifications that could never be caused by the sun or soil, alone. Consequently, nutritional supplementation is more important than it has ever been. But if we depend on avaricious minds to supply us with nutrients, we will only get active ingredients opposed to all the ingredients provided by nature. In terms of nature's medicines, herbs are not thoroughly safe because plants are being controlled for profit. It is common for Big Pharma mentalities to refine or over-process herbs and nutritional supplements to the point that the nutrients are removed. They are destroying life and definitely doing harm.

The health food industry should not be trusted. Surely, it earns money, but only because Big Food has frightened the public. Most people do not know the difference between organic and inorganic produce. However, the idea of eating pure, clean, chemical-free food is merely a fantasy created by marketers that could not imagine eating healthy food for any reason. Money is the mission and motivation. And consumers in need of organic produce and products are unknowingly collecting inorganic toxins with every mouthful.

The next time you eat a candy bar and feel energetic, remember that you are ingesting an isolated concentrate in the form of extracted sugar. Yes, the body will be excited by the intrusion of the poison and the body will react to remove it. This will be misconstrued as energy or a "feel-good", but the body is degenerating while the pancreas, liver and kidney are weakened. The body will only provide a reactionary defense until it is no longer nutritionally able. At that time, it will submit to the drugs, such as sugar, that we see as harmless.

Unfortunately, Mexico has an obesity issue. And type 2 diabetes is listed as the leading killer. In Mexico, soft drinks are cheaper than water. And of course, the soda industry would like for the people to believe that there is no link between obesity and the poisons they bottle. Like any other poison, carbonated drinks can become addictive. Sure, the beverage may make you feel better until the body develops a tolerance. At this point, the body requires more of the substance to get the feeling that it experienced initially. The body has to maintain homeostasis or an ideal state of health by neutralizing any detrimental or foreign substances. The effects of foodstuffs and drugs are gradually minimized as the body learns to mitigate them. However, the average eater is addicted to taste and the idea of eating without understanding the purpose of food or being satiated. Due to the lack of satisfaction, more food than is necessary is consumed by the individual. And though the body knows that the substances lack nutrition, it develops a new level of tolerance and craves more toxic substances.

Our demand for food forces our bodies to a range of functioning that the body is encouraged to endure. Unfortunately, the body goes into a mode of self-protection and adjusts to substances of choice and the damages that accompany them. Certainly, the body will react over a period of time. Hunger pains, headaches, acne, flatulence, infrequent bowel movements, insomnia, joint aches and other symptoms are signs of the body's need to withdraw from the damaging practices.

Modern medicine considers an ailment to be an often persistent bodily disorder or disease; a cause for complaining. As the body no longer functions as intended, we habitually seek relief. No time is given for the body to make corrections because we are programmed to find care immediately. Usually, we find comfort in drugs. If OTC drugs or a friend's suggestion does not work, we visit the doctor. Medical doctors have the privilege of experimentation. If the first drug does not work, you are given another drug with an excuse that suggests your body needs something stronger. Regardless, the drug cannot heal the body and the presence of the drug is only complicating the process of healing. Problems are being compounded with the food stuffs and the prescription drugs. Each drug remains in the body for a certain amount of time. Every poison is different.

In *The Alcoholism Addiction Cure*, Chris Prentiss explains the duration of drug's effects and the meaning of "half-life". Half-life refers to the length of time it takes for the drug to reach 50 percent of its original potency. Depending on the medication prescribed, the half-life could range from two to six days. This means that that if you take a pill with a half-life of three days, the concentration will decrease by 50 percent every three days until the drug is no longer in the body. However, it has been stated that seven half-lives will sufficiently rid the body of almost all effects of a toxin. Mathematically speaking, this formula is applied to each pill that is taken. So, if an individual is taking multiple pills each day and it takes seven half-lives to get it out of the system, one's system will have to contain and entertain the toxin for weeks to several months. Moreover, if one complains to the physician about the prescription and receives a different prescription, they will only exacerbate the problem because physicians sell drugs and they do not mind stacking one drug on top of another. Therefore, it can take several months to cleanse the body of poisons. And foodstuffs do not facilitate the process of detoxification. This is the reason that most rehabilitation centers for drugs are failures and anonymous associations to deal with addictions are in business. Such companies merely provide an opportunity for people with addictions to swap addictions. And in all irony, the majority of individuals suffering from an addiction will choose a malnutritious foodstuff or sexual activity to satisfy their needs.

The big pharmaceutical companies work hard to offer drugs around the world at prices that people cannot afford or variations that the body does not need. However, physicians have convinced their patients that an unnatural product, which will be recognized as a poison, will save their life or buy them time. These companies do not care to offer low-cost versions of the poisons because emphasis is placed on chemicals opposed to human lives. Of course, Big Pharma spends billions of dollars on TV ads that exaggerate the industry's so-called virtue and compassion. But the truth is – drugs do not and cannot cure. There are no good drugs! Drugs are basically addictive and can easily modify one's behavior. Surely, drugs distract the brain when one is in pain, but it doesn't cure anything. An individual can be isolated from the drug of choice and immediately return to experiencing the previous feelings and pains. The body's method of alarming you to the issue that you wish to ignore is switched off. It can be schizophrenia, depression, toothache, back pain, headache or any ailment, the body wants your attention to what is happening or on the verge of happening. To ignore the warning is an attitude equivalent to placing electrical tape over a check engine indicator of car that is already smoking. I must admit, it would be better to disrobe for a clueless stranger in a white coat than to have him place his nasty stethoscope against you, take your temperature, check your reflexes and give you a prescription without determining your body's imbalance than to continue ignoring the body.

The fact that the disease industry wants to use a drug to cure every physical and mental condition without discovering why energy is being held, what caused an ailment or why the immune system is compromised, is every reason for holistic practitioners to recognize Nature and listen to the body. Of course, some alternative health practitioners do not have the ability to determine what is happening with a client. They simply use the information that they are given by the sickly individual or they make the mistake of treating the person as they did another person with the same ailments based on misinformation.

Psychologists do not refer to chemistry when determining chemical or brain imbalances in individuals. Their billing bible, *Diagnostic and Statistical Manual of Mental Disorders*, which is intended to diagnose, label and bill, has a minimum of 374 mental disorders that defines every human life on the planet: anybody can be labeled with a mental disorder. The dispensary of drugs is motivated by perks that honest healing cannot offer. The pseudo-science is actually managing questionable illnesses with drugs because they cannot cure the questionable illnesses. And drugs are being prescribed to qualify persons that would not count as doctors. It is known that doctors must have patients.

I love Mexico, but the average work schedule interferes with the concept of proper living. The commonality seems normal, but most folks are stressed. Life in Mexico is much slower than life in the U.S., but there are issues which are accepted as the norm that make for stressful news in the U.S., as well. And stress is always accompanied by addictions.

The disease industry does not want living or healing to be simplified and this blatant fact will never be erased with the truth or a little, white lie. Most of our illnesses can be corrected with rest, sufficient amounts of water, sunlight, proper nutrition, exercise, clean air, proper breathing, and positive thoughts. It isn't as simple as walking five flights of stairs, eating a pork chop sandwich with light mayonnaise accompanied by a trendy jar of salad and praying on Sunday. There are reasons for the body to offer pain, signs and symptoms. Our response to said indicators is germane. And too, an objective assessment of one's ability to function should be observed before they are subjected to poisons.

Culture speaks volumes. Carnitas, tortillas, salsa and nopales immediately paint a picture of Mexico. Just as hotdogs, baseball, apple pie, neuroticism and racism paint a picture of the United States. Of course, the two comparisons are not equivalent. Nonetheless, the newer generations have to find alternatives to replace the accepted foods and traditions that are abbreviating our lives with pain and imbalance without complicating and modernizing life with convenient synthetics. It is possible for people to define happiness holistically and too, experience it without foodstuffs and toxins that alter one's biochemistry. Living is accompanied by a level of wisdom and strength, but living strong and not improving one's conditions should never be preferred over living properly and applying common sense.

Often I hear people refer to themselves as being healthy simply because they do not wear glasses, lack a pot belly, lead a vegetarian lifestyle, eat organic foods or find themselves to be attractive. Seriously? Today, the soils aren't anything like what they used to be. Of course, poor quality foods cannot possibly sustain a high level of health without one consuming an abundance of the selected food to meet what Nature intended. Our soils yield plants with inadequate amounts of phosphorous, calcium and trace minerals. In addition, the soils lack microbial balance and the carbon cycling is extremely poor. The carbon cycle is defined as the continuous process by which carbon is exchanged between organisms and the environment. Carbon dioxide is absorbed from the atmosphere by plants and algae and converted to carbohydrates by photosynthesis. Carbon is then passed into the food chain and returned to the atmosphere by the respirations and decay of animals, plants, and other organisms.

Still, we mimic the importance of organic foods without testing what we have been convinced to believe. The Organic Trade Association released the results of the U.S Families Organic Attitudes and Beliefs Study conducted in January of 2013 to show that 81% of families   purchase some organic items. We want to believe that anything that grows or lives on Earth was provided for our consumption by the most merciful God. We would also like to believe that such a large percentage of people believe in government certified produce when it is possible that only 100 people were interviewed on cold an extremely cold day while wearing mittens. How is it that a people that strategically choose to eat the less aggressive animals have become so aggressive about their health during the struggles of the current U.S. administration? Consequently, people don't go to butchers or grocers to pick up freshly murdered tiger, elephant, lion, wolf, jaguar or bear. And individuals that eat alligator weren't thrilled with its consumption until they saw people wrestling, kissing and controlling them.

Organic gardening places its focus on input. Yes, nitrogen, phosphorous and potassium or NPK. Some gardeners add sulfur, as well. However, this particular addition is expected to give the plants and soil better nutrition even though most plants do not have the same nutrient requirements.

Dr. Keith Moreno

When we hear the word organic, our minds waver. For the most part, we visualize a tie-dyed T-shirt wearing person with unkempt hair hugging a tree to save it, or chaining themselves to a building to prevent the masses from losing jobs, or a radical person eating granola and fruit mixes sprinkled with seeds while sipping on wheatgrass. Some people that fit the definition of organic carry incense to deodorize their presence. The word "organic" is often very misused and misleading. It can imply that something is without chemicals or preservatives. But that perception is based on the government's idea of what amount of chemicals and preservatives is safe and allowable.

Organic is a term previously used to describe a molecule bound by a chain of carbon atoms. Surely, the term is used nowadays as a marketing strategy to promote something that would never be recognized as healthy. And then the confusion increases when Big Pharma offers drugs that permit organic sex or society suggests organic sex as if "raw" makes it better. Organic sex is supposedly performed without any type of protection. This whole concept is thought to be organic or so damn original. It is obvious that organic is no longer organic. And organic stuff is not necessarily the best. Besides, modern agriculturists are routinely producing an enormous amount of low-quality foods that are preserved with added colors, gases, genetic modification, irradiation, and waxes that cannot improve the nutritional value. Other so-called foods are subjected to extreme processing, contamination and harmful preservatives.

I encourage a diet that is absent of animal flesh and animal by-products, but I am aware of the poor grade of produce and even more skeptical of companies offering nutraceuticals. I understand that need to eat more fruits and vegetables than any government may suggest that people eat. An exceptional idea is to eat a piece of fruit (prior to 2pm) or selected vegetable (that can be eaten without cooking) every 30 minutes until 7pm each day. Of course, water is extremely important, but somehow downplayed.

The people are experiencing mineral deficiencies because the soil is deficient in minerals and cannot meet the nutrient requirements of the produce that will eventually be overcooked. Nonetheless, there is a way to have your medicines in the form of food. And too, this method empowers the consumer and the grower because both focus on the results of the plants. A plant-based diet is a beautiful concept, but if the produce lacks in nutrients, the recipients' health will be questionable.

Most raw foodists, chefs and health gurus promise a life of eternity without ever offering a solution. Sure, you can grow your own food and you can be your own doctor, but if you lack knowledge about soil and the needs of the body, you are not any more progressive than you were with your physician and his/her superstitions.

Get Serious About Living Properly!

In all likelihood, your choice of doctor, diet and medications has not improved your health. So, imagine if you could test nutrient levels in selected produce before you purchase or in the produce that you grow in your garden. As you decide to grow the plants in 5 gallon buckets, pots, empty milk jugs, paint cans, or in areas that were previously saved for roses or ferns, you could add organic matter to the soil and continue to test to get the results that promise more nutrients. Undoubtedly, foliar feeding (spraying fertilizers to leaves) and manure teas will improve productivity. You don't need a green thumb to grow healthy food.

High Brix produce does not have to be organic because individuals familiar with high brix plants don't care if they are certified to be organic based on the lies and standards of any government's department of agriculture or not. An instrument called a refractometer can make the difference in the produce you buy and your health, in the future. It would be nice to have organic produce grown to high brix standards because high brix foods are superior. Plus, high brix foods do not need protection in the form of insecticides, fungicides, and herbicides.

Reasons High Brix is Better than Trusting Misinformed Farmers, Gurus and Governments:

1.   High Brix produce have greater mineral density.

2.   High Brix produce greater carbohydrate levels, taste.

3.   High Brix foods are insect and disease resistant.

4.   High Brix foods have a richer, better taste.

5.   High Brix foods are instinctively preferred by animals

       that are not overly hungry or close to starvation.

6.   High Brix foods do not rot; it dehydrates.

Is Quality Food Better?

In Mexico City, a fresh foods market can be found each day of the week. And for some reason, inorganic foods grown in the U.S. are available as well. Why? In the U.S., produce is grown cheaply and sold for 3 times the amount it cost to grow and harvest. However, seeking out cheap or bad vegetables to save money is not recommended. Consequently, buying food just to eat in order to prevent hunger or starvation may eventually prove to be an expensive decision.

Produce that looks good and seems to keep well, while in the stores, due to the saturation of chemicals and the periodic water sprays, is in reality graded poorly in terms of actual food value. You cannot expect to improve nutrition with a low nutritional quality. Again, you cannot trust the seller or the appearance of food. Quality will be more expensive. In Mexico, salesmen volunteer samples of produce. It is easier to test the quality without sampling for taste. As the health improves and one lives properly, there are no extra expenses for overrated insurance, low grade nutritional supplements, medications and the purchase of nutrient-poor foods.

Seasonal Foods

Nature knows best and Nature and has proven that all foods cannot be eaten every day, week or month. There are times of day and times of year for foods to be eaten. Canned and frozen foods are excellent for survival situations such as a political uprising, power outages or when travel is prohibited due to iced roads or roadblocks. Otherwise, having knowledge of what foods are in season is advisable. In addition, look for foods that are locally grown. Support the Farmer´s Markets. The following lists are seasonal produce. Mind you, the lists are not complete and more importantly, some produce is shipped from other regions and countries.

Spring	Summer	Autumn	Winter
March	June	September	December
April	July	October	January
May	August	November	February

Spring Produce (List for U.S.)

Asparagus	Green garlic	Peas
Apricots	Grapefruit	Pineapple
Artichoke	Kohlrabi	Radishes
Arugula	Kumquats	Rhubarb
Beets	Lemons	Scallions
Carrots	Leeks	Spinach
Chard (greens)	Mangoes	Strawberries
Cherries	Nettles	Turnips
Fava beans	Navel Oranges	
Fennel	Parsley	

Summer

Apples	Carrots	Eggplant
Avocados	Chard	Strawberries
Apricots	Corn	Peaches
Blackberries	Cherries	Tomatoes
Boysenberries	Chiles	Basil
Cantaloupe	Cucumbers	Blueberries

Autumn

Apples	Eggplant	Wild Mushrooms	Rapini
Artichokes	Fennel	Okra	Radishes
Arugula	Figs	Onions	Rutabaga
Beets	Garlic	Parsnips	Scallions
Broccoli	Grapes	Pears	Shallots
Brussel Sprouts	Green Beans	Persimmons	Shelling Beans
Carrots	Kale	Peppers	Sweet Potatoes
Cauliflower	Kohlrabi	Pumpkins	Turnips
Celery	Leeks	Potatoes	Winter Squash
Cabbage	Lemongrass	Pomegranates	
Cranberries	Limes	Quinces	
Chard	Lettuce	Radicchio	

Winter

Beets	Grapefruit	Papaya
Broccoli	Artichoke	Pomelos
Brussels Sprouts	Kiwi	Potatoes
Cabbage	Kale	Parsnip
Cardoons	Kohlrabi	Watermelon
Carrots	Kumquats	Winter Squash
Cauliflower	Lemons	Tangerines
Celery	Leeks	Shallots
Clementines	Mandarins	Rutabaga
Escarole	Onions	Sweet Potatoes
Fennel	Oranges	Tangelos

List taken, in part, from *this foodthing.com*

The following lists are sectioned into months for produce in Mexico. Whether visiting or living in Mexico, this is information that is normally taken for granted. We never assume that restaurants serve foods that aren't in season, even if fast food

ENERO

Verduras: Calabacitas, col, coliflor, chiles poblanos, espinacas, hongos, lechuga, papas, zanahorias.

Frutas: Fresas, guayabas, jícamas, limas, limón, mandarina, naranja, papaya, piña, plátano, toronja, uva.

FEBRERO

Verduras: Calabacitas, col, coliflor, chiles poblanos, espinacas, hongos, lechuga, papas, zanahorias, berenjena.

Frutas: Fresas, guayabas, limas, limón, mandarina, mamey, melón, naranja, papaya, piña, plátano, toronja, uva.

MARZO

Verduras: Alcachofas, calabacitas, col, coliflor, espinacas, hongos, lechuga, nopales, papas, pepinos, tomates, jitomates.

Frutas: Fresa, limón, mandarina, melón, naranja, papaya, piña, plátano, sandia, toronja.

ABRIL

Verduras: Calabacitas, coliflor, ejotes, espinacas, hongos, lechugas, nopales, papas, pepinos, tomates, jitomates, zanahorias.

Frutas: Fresa, limón, mango, melón, mamey, naranja, papaya, pera, piña, plátano, sandia, toronja.

MAYO

Verduras: Calabacitas, coliflor, chiles poblanos, ejotes, elotes, espinacas, hongos, lechuga, nopales, papas, pepinos, tomates, jitomates, zanahorias.

Frutas: Ciruela, chabacano, durazno, limón, mango, melón, papaya, piña.

JUNIO

Verduras: Calabacitas, durazno, coliflor, chiles poblanos, ejotes, elotes, espinacas, hongos, lechuga, nopales, papas, pepinos, tomates, jitomates, zanahorias

Frutas: Ciruela, chabacano, durazno, mango, melón, papaya, pera, espinacas.

JULIO

Verduras: Calabacitas, coliflor, chiles poblanos, ejotes, elotes, hongos, lechuga, papas, pepinos, tomates, berros, jitomates, zanahorias.

Frutas: Ciruela, durazno, limón, mango, manzana, melón, papaya, pera, piña, plátano.

AGOSTO

Verduras: Calabacitas, coliflor, chiles poblanos, ejotes, elotes, hongos, lechuga, papas, pepinos, tomates, jitomates, aguacate, berros, espinacas, zanahorias.

Frutas: Ciruela, durazno, limón, manzana, melón, papaya, pera, piña, plátano, uvas.

SEPTIEMBRE

Verduras: Calabacitas, col, coliflor, chiles poblanos, ejotes, elotes, espinacas, acelgas, hongos, lechuga, papas, pepinos, aguacate, tomates, jitomates, zanahorias.

Frutas: Ciruela, durazno, guayaba, limón, manzana, papaya, pera, plátano, sandia, toronja, uvas.

OCTUBRE

Verduras: Calabacitas, col, chiles poblanos, ejotes, aguacate, espinacas, hongos, lechuga, papas, tomates, jitomates, zanahorias

Frutas: Ciruela, guayaba, lima, limos, mandarina, naranja, manzana, papaya, pera, plátano, toronja, uvas.

NOVIEMBRE

Verduras: Calabacitas, acelga, berenjena, calabaza, col, ejotes, espinacas, hongos, papas, zanahorias.

Frutas: Fresa, guayaba, jícama, lima, limón, mandarina, naranja, papaya, plátano, uvas.

DICIEMBRE

Verduras: Calabacitas, calabaza, col, ejotes, acelga, berenjena, espinacas, hongos, lechuga, papas, zanahorias.

Frutas: Fresa, guayaba, jícama, lima, limón, mandarina, naranja, papaya, piña, plátano, toronja, uva.

Dr. Keith Moreno

How Organic is Organic?

It is believed that organic farming creates richer soil and minimizes pollutants in groundwater and improves our chances of avoiding pesticides in our drinking water. The aspect of minimized chemicals suggests that plant growth will improve and soil erosion will be reduced. Nonetheless, fluoridated water is ruining the soil and altering the produce. It can be argued that not all plants are absorbing fluoride in the same amount, but the truth is that the shortcuts used to rush nature are actually punishing all earthlings.

Organic food doesn't always prove to be better, but it is believed to be healthier due to the absence of fertilizers and pesticides. Without chemicals, plants are able to boost their phytochemical production. Therefore, the plants have the vitamins and antioxidants that strengthen their resistance to weeds and bugs.

Unfortunately, organic food can be grown with approved synthetic ingredients. However, in the U.S. some crops are grown without the use of irradiation, artificial pesticides or synthetic pesticides. Yet, it is safer to assume that a percentage of such crops are certainly genetically modified so that they can withstand the bugs and weeds.

The advantage of the farmer's market is that you can question the farmer or salesperson about where and how the produce was grown. Hopefully, they will have more information than just the cost of the   product. And in terms of health, make it a habit to choose the healthiest of produce by testing it with a *refractometer*.

Milk is really a food. It is a food that is ingested as a drink or eaten in a variety of baked items. Of course, it was intended for a being with four stomachs and four hooves. If you are lactose intolerant and refuse to drink milk, you can always eat your milk. However, 75% of the world is lactose intolerant. Undoubtedly, persons that are melanin dominant are naturally lactose intolerant. According to Dr. Neal Barnard, a clinical researcher, Caucasians have a genetic mutation that allows them to drink and digest milk into adulthood.

The numbers of cheeses found in Mexico are amongst the best kept food secrets of the world. Naturally, some cheeses are more popular than others, but Mexico has Chihuahua, Manchega, Panela, Oaxaca and Blanco to share with the world. Each year, Mexico ranks 10th in the world for cheese production. And it ranks eighth in terms of consumption. However, the United States of America ranks within the top 10 countries with the highest rate for cancer.

Most Mexican cheeses are made from cows' milk despite the fact that milk does nothing good for the body. Of course, milk is one of the most common foods of the modern diet. People drink milk with ease and with almost any type of food. Cow's milk and goat's milk are the most popularly consumed of animal choices. Sheep's milk is preferred by a small percentage. The appeal of animal flesh, bones and fluids is overwhelming. And dairy is definitely liquid meat. It should never be considered a health food.

In the U.S., milk is pasteurized to prevent the somatic cell count from exceeding 750,000 cells/ml. In other words, one glass of milk can have 180 million white blood cells or what should be referred to as pus cells and still be deemed safe to drink. Furthermore, milk is a by-product of blood. The somatic cell count is important because of mastitis. Mastitis is inflammation of the breast and is frequently subclinical or "hidden". The milk farmers would like to hide the fact that the cows have infections that require a heavy use of antibiotics because this is the "goodness" that the people are drinking. The term "somatic" means that it is "derived from the body". All milk derived from animals contains white blood cells known as leukocytes which make up the majority of somatic cells. Somatic cell counts that are higher than 200,000 cells/ml are considered abnormal and indicate probable infection.

Milk has been considered the vitality drink for decades because the intelligence of mankind was arrested and the number of consumers was increased. Meanwhile, the populous has been indoctrinated with pus and lies that allow milk to become a nutritional savior. Milk is miraculously supposed to make the bones strong, build muscles, stop cramps associated with menstruation, increase weight loss, prevent heart disease, improve skin, increase height and strengthen teeth.

There are supposedly two types of proteins found in milk. The most prominent protein is casein; whey protein is the other. Casein represents 80% of the protein in milk, but whey protein is more recognizable. The digestion of a specific type of casein, A1 beta casein, has been found to produce an opioid by-product that can become very problematic for some humans. This particular casein has been associated with autism, schizophrenia, heart disease, diabetes, high cholesterol and a variety of autoimmune disorders. It is believed that the A1 beta casein is a result of a genetic mutation in cattle that possibly occurred around 8,000 years ago in Europe. However, milk remains very popular.

In Mexico, A1 beta casein is very popular. Yes, there is A1 beta casein and A2 beta caseins. Without complicating the issue, I must add that a single amino acid is the big difference between the two. Said difference adds to the already existing problems of milk as if pasteurization did not present enough complications.

Milk is milk, we have been taught. It has been promoted as a   miracle food. And now, raw milk is the trend for would-be health conscious types. Ironically, any information that is not pleasing to the ear is considered not to be trustworthy. Raw milk, which comes straight from the udder of a cow is said to be a complete and balanced food. This theory is based on cow-udder-calf logic and the fact that the calf becomes a part of the adult cattle population if it is not slaughtered to meet the demands for veal. Humans love milk, but cows, heifers, stags, bulls, and oxen do not drink it after childhood. Raw milk does not need to be enriched with vitamins or minerals. And too, as it ferments, the taste and benefits are said to improve. Raw milk is categorized as a living food with protective properties. Perhaps, this implies that raw milk is better for human consumption than milk produced or stolen from cows that are strategically fed antibiotics and genetically modified crops that offer hormone-contaminated milk.

A many people are under the impression that everything that God made is good and that anything that is bad was made by his creation, the devil. Interesting! God is merciful and beneficent and his creation is equally horrific, but Nature plays by a different set of rules. Consequently, governments and businesses just do as they wish without any model of consciousness or conscience.

Sweet Milk?

We cannot escape the concept of durational suicide or the chemicals that are added and hidden in our foods. This is the reason that any food that is packaged should be avoided. The need to use every substance, whether safe or not, makes the science of doing business somewhat difficult. The business of providing cheap foods becomes an art that offers a slow death. In the U.S., the Food and Drug Administration has been asked to approve of aspartame being added to milk. To ask for approval signifies that sweeteners are already being used to alter the taste of pus and blood. Try to imagine what lurks in chocolate milk. Furthermore, if it is disapproved, the aspartame will be added because the International Dairy Foods Association and National Milk Producers Federation only want to gauge the reactions of the people and of course, verify what amount of poison can be added without being detected by consumers. This is cleverly accomplished without placing the petition on *Facebook* to be recognized by the distracted and trusting public that will actually be affected by the consumption of this poison. This isn't proper or fair!

Aspartame causes damage to the body and yet, these organizations are labeling it and other additives as "safe and suitable". Mind you, aspartame was thoroughly studied before its approval in 1981. Of course, animals and willing humans were giving the poison in amounts considered to be greater than what the average person would consume in their diet. The chosen subjects were eventually diagnosed with diabetes, special genetic conditions, and obesity. However, these studies were never made public record.

If consciousness, intelligence or some type of enlightenment has changed your way of life and you feel fortunate, think again. Milk derivatives are in foods that do not require milk. And too, products do not require plain language on the label. Milk derivatives can be labeled as vegetable fat, hydrolyzed whey protein, sodium caseinate, calcium caseinate, margarine and the list goes on.

Foodstuffs continue to affect people. Some people are not damaged as quickly as others. In addition, aspartame reacts with all drugs, vaccines and/or toxic substances. In the U.S., millions of people are affected by aspartame. And for the mothers that do not know the effects that aspartame can have on children, they should be informed that mother's milk is preferred over cow's pus-filled, mucus forming milk and that aspartame contains 10 percent free methanol which is a neurotoxin. As aspartame metabolizes in the body, additional methanol is created. Aspartame is an excitotoxin and it is likely already in your milk and other dairy products without your knowledge or consent. Surely, there will be an increase in cases of epileptic seizures, diabetes, erratic child behavior and visual damage and doctors will misdiagnose and compound another problem. Besides, milk does a lot of good for business!

The fact that we expect "dead" alkaline water to clean up the poisons sold by food and drug companies is embarrassing. We don't realize that it is produced by heat and therefore, a drug. Confusion abounds due to our inability to determine whether alkaline products are beneficial or dangerous. Some of us would just like to know how to make the "best water" without buying a machine or having to make monthly purchases of packets of solvents that promise to do what the body naturally does. Most consumers of alkaline water and products do not know if drinking alkaline water makes the body alkaline or not. They simply trust the marketing of minds that convince us that weight loss, without exercise, is not only possible - but also healthy and long-term. Unfortunately, alkaline water does not make the body alkaline. It cannot make this change. And the thought, alone, ignores the process of digestion.

The popular abbreviation that copy and paste practitioners habitually use to sell meaningless products is known as pH. It stands for Potential Hydrogen and oftentimes means nothing more than high profits. The pH scale is likened to a chemical measuring stick that determines if a substance is alkaline or acidic. The left side of the pH scale measures the presence of dominant hydrogen atoms. Remember, hydrogen is known to exist in large concentrations in acids. Moreover, the hydrogen atoms exist in molecules. And on the right side of the scale are the dominant alkalis. Naturally, the presence of dominant substances speaks to absence of opposites.

The pH scale has a neutral zone as well. Understandably, a pH of 7.0 is not acid or alkaline; it is the point of balance or calm. In addition, we must note that alkalis dissolve matter and acids burn matter.

The Emphasis of Hydrogen

According to the periodic table, hydrogen is the lightest gas that man has discovered. It has no smell, color or taste. Perhaps, it is most comparable to the most celebrated mythological characters in our minds that we have not seen or cannot prove to have existed. Yet, it is very common and undoubtedly, extremely important because hydrogen atoms are the building blocks of life. Plus, this powerful element that is at the core of all life makes up 90% of the atoms of the universe.

Man or what man now refers to as the "human being" is a carbon based organism consisting of acids, fats, enzymes, proteins and carbohydrates. Our bones are a combination of carbon and hydrogen or what are called hydrocarbons. Furthermore, hydrogen is found in vegetables, fruits, meats and component parts such as amino acids and sugars. Without hydrogen, acids would not have potential energy.

The human body is capable of converting hydrogen through the process of extracting energy with the action of metabolism. Human digestion works like a furnace with hydrogen that serves as the combustible substance. As the hydrogen burns, it releases heat and energy. This conversion feeds the carbon based organism. Contrary to what we are taught about acids, live acids supply energy that progresses organic life.

The Hype of Alkali

An alkali can easily be remembered as a base. Yet, it is a corrosive element that is used as a solvent because it dissolves matter. Alkalis are found in glass, detergents, and the farming industry and in various types of sodium. Food-based alkalis interfere with human metabolism and too, absorb acids. And despite being told that an alkaline body is healthy, most life on earth prefers a pH level of 7.0 which is neither alkaline nor acid. In addition, cells that are loaded in hydrogen are commonly alive, unless the acid content is so great that the cells completely lack complex life.

As a rule, when an alkali becomes active, it melts matter and as a result, creates a mild alkaline slime. However, when acid is released, it burns and leaves behind alkali ash residue. A fire burns within the body. The solar plexus is proof of the light within. Of course, there is no actual flame in the body, but the existing heat offers vaporization and the same results as a flame. The human body digests matter by utilizing a strong acid to release energy for the purpose of maintenance and healing. Once the acid of the stomach is weakened, digestion becomes sluggish and the body suffers.

When equal amounts of acid and alkali coexist in the body, we experience equilibrium, balance or homeostasis. However, the partnership of science and business gives the industry ample reason to produce solvents. And again, the question should be whether or not the people are to trust administrations responsible for overseeing foods and drugs. Alkalis are corrosive and destitute of much needed life giving energy. However, they are equipped with life dissolving energy.

Alkalis can be made by burning something in a fire or in a laboratory. Consequently, cooking is a source that produces alkalis. Most foods that are cooked easily become alkaline unless the cooking process is able to release the latent acidic components that make the mixture more acidic and therefore, more potent.

When alkaline products are consumed, the immune system is alerted and attempts to destroy the invader. Naturally, digestion converts the alkaline to an acid. Alkaline water does not prevent disease, cure disease or protect anyone from a disorder. Furthermore, the drugs camouflaged as nutritional supplements and processed foods are responsible for suppressing digestion. Anything eaten, at this stage, will simply layer in the stomach causing blockage in the colon and the buildup of gases. Hydrochloric acid, which is very necessary, becomes limited and indigestion is the result. Yes, the indigestion is caused by too little acid opposed to too much acid. Nonetheless, indigestion is the accumulation of alkaline foods or liquids lacking enzymes that cannot digest at the same speed as live acids.

Acid Body Theory

Anybody with a pH product to sell will tell you that cancers thrive in bodies with too much acid. This is part of the sales pitch. Like parrots, they have learned to repeat stuff that sounds scientific, intelligent or impressionable. They will also go against Nature and say that acidic foods, provided by nature, contribute to an acidic environment as well. And let's not forget that cancers gain momentum in oxygen depleted environments. I dutifully accept the theory that cancer is caused by an accumulation of acidic waste that builds over a period of time due to lifestyle, thoughts, diet and chemical residue. And more importantly, I acknowledge that the immune system is not properly functioning. Yet, why the immune system has failed is rarely addressed.

When considering what foods to eat, people should find a balance between fruits, vegetables, proteins and starches, if they are not addicted to such foods. It is not a good idea to shock the system with a diet, new method of eating or product that will only worsen the condition without the person's knowledge. Really, we have to learn to eat foods in a manner that does not generate toxins. But this is difficult because food fills so many voids. Perhaps, the use of microwaves, stoves, hot plates and generators has served its purpose. For persons that must have meat, thinly sliced raw meats or fermented meats will offer the greatest nutritional benefit due to live enzymes and protein concentrations. In addition, dehydrated herbs, which are considered mild alkalinic, medicinal substances, are referred to as foods. And they have medicinal properties that can assist the body in detoxification and raising the pH level.

To summarize, alkaline water and products do not and cannot alkalize the body because chemistry of the human body and Nature suggest that it is impossible. The digestive sequence works as follows: a live acidic food is eaten; live acid fuel is extracted via digestion; digestion lets the body use the acid fuel to make heat and heal; the digestive tract uses any available acids from the food; and acids used in the digestive process result in alkaline waste. Again, the conversion from acid fuel converts to alkaline waste. The over-priced, useless alkaline products are assumed to be ingested and unchanged by the body. If this notion is true, said product actually had very little effect on the body. Furthermore, anything not utilized by the body will pass through the body in the same form as it entered: for example, kernels of corn, poorly chewed nuts or a penny with a hole in it. If alkaline products are to cause change, they must mix with another component in order to create a new substance. The mixture dilutes the solution until it is eventually so weak that it no longer resembles the original form.

Remember, alkaline water is produced by heat and it is definitely dead. Once the toxin is consumed, the body attacks it. Naturally, digestion converts the alkaline to the opposite. In this case, it becomes an acid. Alkaline water and products should be recognized as a drug because the detoxification reaction is nothing more than the body's rejection of a mild poison.

Cancer is an industry that rakes in hundreds of millions of dollars each year in the U.S., and nothing less than a billion dollars, globally. It is estimated by the more significant research agencies that more than four trillion dollars have been donated to cancer research since being recognized as a problem. What is the money for? If it is for research to find a cure, it would be better for scientists to share the cause of the disease that has become an industry. Ironically, a large number of people would lose jobs, if a cure is ever promoted.

The face of cancer is changing so much that we are learning that there are alternatives to chemotherapy and radiation. Once cancer has been detected, it should be dealt with immediately. Cancer is cancer. And panic will only create more stress.

The cause of cancer can be linked to chemicals, radiation and viruses. Consequently, vaccinations are a popular method for transferring viruses. And too, there are not any guidelines to verify that the vaccines are toxin-free.

There is no way for a person diagnosed with cancer to continue with the same toxic lifestyle because their immune system is not working properly. Any and every food that is packaged has to be questioned. All household products and personal cosmetics have to be scrutinized. The individual cannot continue to ingest poisons or apply toxins to the skin, lips and hair.

Nutrition is the most practical, intelligent and economical way to address cancer after detoxification. This idea is frowned upon because soil, chlorophyll and nutrition are not properly understood. However, obtaining the proper nutrients will prevent malnutrition and improve immune functions. The cancer cannot be starved via fasting, but the cancer can be starved by avoiding sugar.

The disease industry is capable of speaking fear into patients. The patients of the disease industry are convinced that if they do not accept the radiation and chemotherapy that they will die. And if a child is diagnosed with cancer and the parents decide to use an alternative, they are charged with neglect. It is important that the individual, diagnosed with cancer, not see the diagnosis as a death sentence because with immediate and necessary changes, it is not.

Big Pharma and the disease industry have notoriously taken half-truths and persuaded the public to sacrifice their health. Rebecca Carley, M.D. stated in Inoculations: Weapons of Mass Destruction that "The basic truth that served as the foundation for the mountain of lies known as vaccinations was the observation that mammals which recover from infection with microorganisms acquire natural immunity from further infections. Whenever cytotoxic T cells (the little Pac man cells which devour and neutralize viruses, bacteria, and cancer cells, thus conferring cellular immunity and are also responsible for allograft rejection) and B cells (antibody producing cells which confer humoral immunity by circulating in the body's fluids or "humors", primarily serum or lymph) are activated by various substances foreign to the body called antigens, some of the T and B cells become memory cells. Thus, the next time the individual meets up with that same antigen, the immune system can be quickly triggered to demolish it. This is the process known as natural immunity."

This is how the vaccination theory was birthed and popularized. Supposedly, a foreign antigen was supposed to be injected into an individual and that antigen would make the individual immune to any infections in the future. However, Dr. Carley explains that the promoters of vaccinations failed to realize that secretory Immunoglobulin A (IgA) that is found in saliva and secretions of the respiratory and gastrointestinal tract mucosa is the initial normal antibody response to all ingested and airborne pathogens.

Everybody has an idea of what a cold may or may not be. But when accumulated mucus is forced from the body, it is because IgA protects the body from viral infections, neutralizes microbial toxins, agglutinates bacteria and decreases the attachment of pathogens to mucosal surfaces. However, when an organism (vaccination) and adjuvants (substances that stimulate the immune system and increases the response) are injected into the body, it causes eventual corruption in the immune system and the IgA is transformed into IgE (an isotype that plays an essential role in allergies) and/or the B cells are hyperactivated to produce pathological, self-attacking antibodies and suppress the cytotoxic T cells.

Everything is being influenced by machinery and chemicals. And the pathogenic viruses that are injected into the body cannot be eliminated by the immune system and therefore, remain in the body. It should be clear that when antigens are surrounded by antibodies the result is serum sickness that spirals into a chronic infection which reproduces and mutates as the sickened body is exposed to more toxins and antigens.

The disease industry has monopolized terms, claimed the color of white and established itself as "all-knowing". Natural medicine is now considered an alternative when the youth, inexperience, record of wrongful deaths, misdiagnoses, improper use of medications, surgical removal of healthy or wrong organs/appendages and medical mistakes of the disease industry prove that said industry of medicine should be the alternative or last resort.

The colon is referred to as the large intestine. The ileum (last part of the small intestine) connects to the cecum (first part of the colon) in the lower right abdomen. The rest of the colon is divided into four parts:

1.   Ascending colon: travels up the right side.

2.   Transverse colon: moves horizontally across the

        abdomen.

3.   Descending colon: runs down the left side.

4.   Sigmoid colon: short curved section (before the rectum).

The colon is responsible for absorbing the remaining water and electrolytes from indigestible food matter; accepting and storing food remains that were not digested in the small intestine; and of course, eliminating solid waste from the body. Today, the process of elimination is complicated due to processed foods and the fact that the body is not performing as it is supposed to perform. Therefore, the skin is considered a part of the elimination system. However, it should not be. This is not to say that sweat isn't necessary or that the body's largest organ cannot eliminate waste. The skin is not the preliminary method of cleansing and should not be treated as such.

The colon works to maintain the body's fluid balance. It absorbs certain vitamins, and processes indigestible material (such as fiber), and stores waste before it is eliminated. Within the colon, the mixture of fiber, small amounts of water, and vitamins, and other things mix with mucus and the bacteria that live in the large intestine, to initiate the formation of solid waste.

The colon has over one hundred trillion microorganisms (bacteria). There are more microorganisms in the colon than are in all other parts of the body combined. A proper balance of healthy bacteria must be maintained inside the colon to avoid being constantly plagued with digestive ailments that eventually contribute to dis-ease.

Environmental Toxins

Planetary pollution should be a concern for the people. Ironically, environmental toxins are a concern for animals and plant-life. Toxins are in the foods that we eat because we normally choose to eat processed foods or cover our foods with additives and preservatives that damage our bodies. Of course, vegetarians must be concerned because a meatless diet heavy in sugar and carbohydrates is not healthy. And each time that I test blood and find heavy metal toxins, I study the sample more thoroughly and hope that there are no signs of cancer. Most cancers are related to environmental factors such as colorings, additives, irradiation, steroids, antibiotics, pesticides, herbicides, dyes, waxes and things that we rarely think of. The manufacturers are contributing to the increase of cancer. Man-made toxins are entering our bodies through the water we drink, the foods we consume, the air we breathe, and the poisonous substances that we apply to our hair, face and skin. The toxins easily find a home in our tissues, fatty cells and vital organs.

We are subjected to an abundance of chemicals. No one is safe, but everyone should want to preserve the planet minus the toxins. Our willful ignorance does nothing to protect us. Accumulated toxins can be presented as dizziness, arthritis, depression, insomnia, allergies, irritability, constipation, indigestion, cold, headache, immune suppression and fatigue. Any of the above indications is proof that the body is suffering. Yet, low energy is enough of an indicator to know that the body needs to be cleansed. The detoxification process targets the skin, intestines, kidney, liver, joints, heart and lungs. Undoubtedly, the use of raw (fresh) produce, exercise, water, colonics, massages, enemas and lymphatic drainage are helpful in eliminating toxins from the body.

The absence of toxins allows the body to experience more energy and improved health. Detoxification is one of the best healing therapies. However, we refuse to eat on a schedule, fast or drink water. And too, we think nothing of missing a bowel movement when we should actually have two to three bowel movements each day. In simpler terms, we would like to believe that for every meal that is consumed a meal should be eliminated. Yet, this is not happening. So, we are collecting toxins from the environment and simultaneously absorbing toxins from the waste that is putrefying in our colon. Said toxins will gradually enter the blood stream causing you to feel fatigued or sick. Eventually, the intestines are unable to filter food particles or chemicals due to pollution and potential impaction. Moreover, once the intestines are polluted, the possibility of proper absorption of nutrients is minimized. It is common to experience headaches, skin blemishes, nausea, and excessive mucus when the increased levels of toxins have stored in the body or commenced to circulate.

Waste Dumping

During the period of detoxification, in which an individual begins to eliminate waste and break down tissues to remove the garbage, they may feel worse. The discomfort is normally a result of toxins and body obstructions exiting the system. The person may experience diarrhea, pain, muscle cramps, body aches, constipation, body odors, irritability, discharges, rashes, headaches or fatigue. Emotional reactions may occur in the form of fear, anxiety, depression or anger. This occurrence is referred to as retracing.

During the retracing process, the major step of healing is mistaken as a bad thing. However, waste is being discarded and tissues are being renewed. Fortunately, the process usually moves through the body rather quickly so the discomfort factor is brief. The retracing phenomenon happens with touch therapies as well. Consequently, the body may require less food as new tissues are formed and assimilation of ingested food is improved. The increase of fresh, whole foods can remedy this problem and decrease the rate of tissue deterioration. For individuals addicted to flesh and blood, animals raised on a natural diet of grass are the best choice. The grass does not create an acidic environment, and studies have confirmed that there is much less E. coli in grass-fed meat products.

The consumption of whole foods and/or raw foods has been heavily commercialized. Health food stores are no longer places to stop and shop without studying the labels. The same companies that manufacture refined food products have their money and hands in the health food industry. Again, we are forced to read cans, boxes and frozen packages. And too, the health foods are more expensive. Of course, more elaborate lies are used to sell the refined products to people considered to be more intelligent. It is time that we apply rules that save our lives. Terms such as "raw" and "live" foods should be nothing more than "fresh foods"; many of which do not need fire. After all, Dr. Aris Latham of *Sun-Fired Cuisine* has made it clear that Nature has already cooked our foods. Therefore, calling the foods "raw" improperly suggests that they are not cooked or ready to eat.

The ability to differentiate between one feeling bad and retracing is a matter of experience and the individual. In terms of the discomforts experienced, such as skin eruptions, they should not be seen as allergies. However, the body is ridding itself of toxins more quickly than the avenues of urine and fecal matter can handle. Certainly, the possibility of damaged organs should be considered. Normally, the damage is not permanent, but the performance of the organs is not normal. When the body is sick and poor performance of organs without noticeable pain is an indication that we should trust the foods that Nature offers. This means that a greater percentage of our foods should be fresh. And the word "moderation" means nothing to a body that is diseased and continuously entertaining and feeding addictions.

I am certain that we all take in toxins from livestock grown on antibiotics, plants sprayed with herbicides and pesticides, packaged foods that have been heavily processed and refined, or produce that has been labeled "organic". Poor food combining and an abundance of cooked proteins and starches have made our bodies more than filthy. Nature has the solution. Fruits and vegetables are provided year-round. Learning to eat foods in season is the key. In addition, minimizing cooked foods is very important. Plus, fasting or abstaining from food and liquids for a 24 hour period each week will help the body to eliminate toxins. Eating correctly may seem expensive, but it is not as costly as the toxic medications or suggested surgeries that the disease industry thrives on.

Companies with access to laboratories can experiment with chemicals and find ways to steal from Nature without ever acknowledging the debt. Ironically, karma has a way of punishing the consumer. Regardless, marketers tell the consumers what they, the consumer, really want because the consumers don't habitually think of what they need. Therefore, the consumer really doesn't have a "choice" because choice originates with creativity. Unfortunately, people are offered sugar blockers, weekend diets, pills that decrease the feeling of hunger and pills that promise to reduce weight without exercise. Lies are birthed and nurtured with more lies founded on fantasies and the exhaustion of enthusiasm.

European propaganda offers the notion that exercise is good for the heart and lungs. However, pulmonary specialists have proven that cardiovascular exercises, such as running and jumping, only condition the muscles. Should you endure a heart attack, you will learn that strong legs will not improve the condition of your heart. Moreover, exercise does not prevent diseases associated with the heart because heart disease is a systemic disease.

Is exercise necessary? This answer is emphatically "yes". But exercise and a junk food diet will eventually result in a worn out body that once looked very appealing despite the deteriorating organs. Junk food does not qualify as food because it cannot qualify as medicine. Sure, it is comestible, but it robs the body of energy because it has nothing to offer the body. Therefore, foods packaged in cans, bottles, boxes and bags that are frozen, dehydrated, or instant and stored on store shelves for weeks to years is junk based on the fact that it contains high amounts of sugar, sodium, preservatives and bleached white flour. The industry's decision to whiten food items out of the demand for items that suggest beauty, purity and convenience is affecting energy levels, increasing fat, and contributing to fat and gastrointestinal issues.

Exercise is important because it decreases stress and depression. However, it increases creativity, endurance, oxygen supply to cells, flexibility of muscles and bones, and sexual energy. Exercise is also good for improving digestion and self-esteem. And too, it relieves constipation and tension. For individuals hoping to lose fat, exercise is necessary for healthy fat reduction. Understandably, poor dietary intake is the main reason for poor body composition.

By implementing the following exercises, five days per week, for at least 30 minutes each day, an individual will improve flexibility, strengthen the muscle groups that are necessary for daily life, improve the efficiency of the organs and reduce the possibility of injuries. If an individual has been diagnosed with a terminal disease, it is imperative that they exercise a minimum of twice per day. Weight-lifting or the desire to be weighed down with muscle built on junk foods, protein shakes and damaging supplements is non-essential. It is possible to have a sexy, healthy body with calisthenics and nutrient-dense foods. The body requires movement. Diets and persons advocating nutrition without exercise are not logical or holistic. The body needs functional exercises that develop cardiovascular endurance, muscular endurance, balance, flexibility, coordination, speed and muscular strength. In addition, an individual desiring to improve their health does not need the latest equipment, a celebrity trainer, an over-priced gadget that promises a body that fitness models wouldn't dare to use at home or machines that isolate parts of the body.

Exercises

The following exercises are utilized and suggested by Dr. Moreno. There are no charts with cycles of exercises or number of repetitions. The important thing is that the individual become motivated by the idea of increased creativity and better health. If you can do a variety of high-intensity exercises for a set period of time and rest for a period of 30 to 60 seconds and then perform another group of exercises, you can burn more calories, build more muscle and increase the metabolism.

Prostration Exercise.

This exercise is recommended for persons that have been diagnosed with cancer. Of course, this exercise, alone, will not cure cancer.

1) Start in the standing position. 2) Kneel and place hands on floor. 3) Immediately begin to crawl until your body is completely extended. 4) Reverse the position until on your knees. 5) Return to standing position.

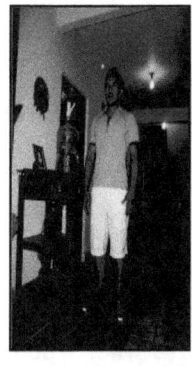 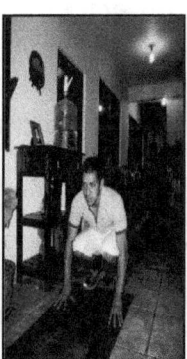 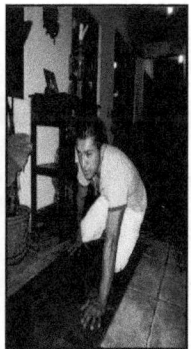 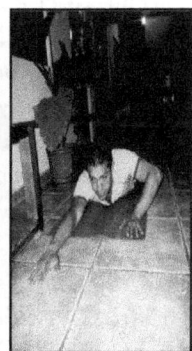

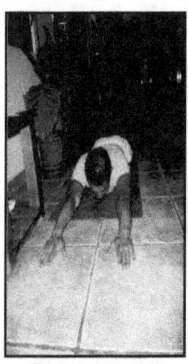 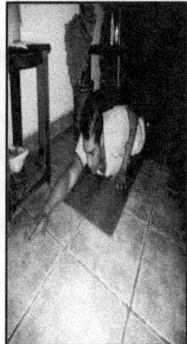 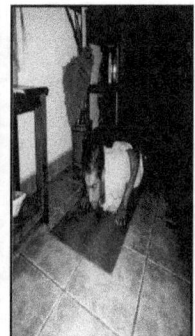 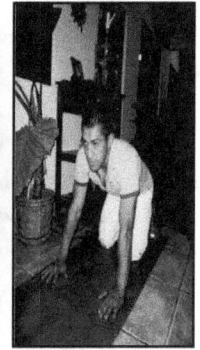

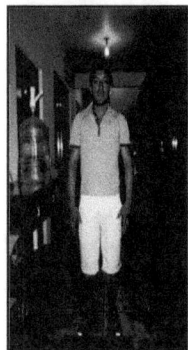

Repeat the exercise a minimum of **30 times**. If you do not find this exercise to be beneficial, you should consider using a number of the beneficial exercises on the following pages in order to   strengthen the core, improve mobility and stimulate your immune system.

Body weight exercises are recommended over the use of weights, exercise gadgets or machines because overall muscle mass and the core are not utilized with the majority of the aforementioned. Bodyweight exercises are safer and actually build more realistic and lasting strength. And too, there are more functional exercises that resemble day-to-day activities. However, there are a number of exercise programs that appear to be functional and effective when in actuality they are useless.

The following exercises are not designed to build the body of a bodybuilder, but actually to make the person fit and strong. And if you are over-weight or unhappy with what the mirror reveals when you are naked, you will have to reduce caloric intake and prepare to burn more calories than you ingest. You should not expect to remove five years of fat gain in five weeks. However, building muscle is one of the best ways to burn fat.

If you do not wish to do exercises, it is important that you incorporate *fasting, colonic irrigations* and *massages* into your life. In addition, if you are aging, gaining weight, have tried diet pills and sense that you unhealthy, detoxification is necessary. Refer to chapter *What We Eat and Think*.

For persons desiring routines, they should select two or three exercises and do each one for one minute and then rest for one minute. Consider doing three sets of each exercise and up to 15 repetitions of each exercise. This is the fastest way to strengthen the body and reduce the fat.

Other Beneficial Exercises

The following exercises are recommended for persons that would like to improve their health, strength and physique. Mind you, there are a number of ways to burn the fat and gain strength without the use of weights.

Calisthenics are definitely easier on the joints. Plus, they offer a plethora of exercises ranging from plyometric to static exercises. Resistance bands are a wonderful addition for persons afraid of suffering weight-related injuries and are not looking for the body builder type body.

Classic Push-up

Chest, Shoulders, Triceps and Core

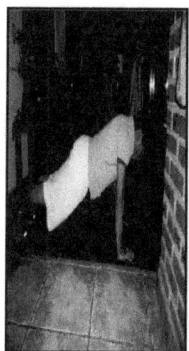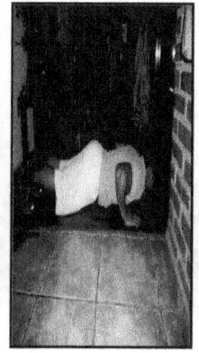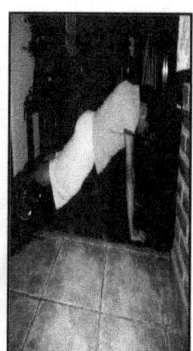

Start in the plank position. Keep the core tight. Be sure to breathe. Slower movements will build more strength. Number of repetitions is not important. Move slowly for 30 to 60 seconds. If you do not do any other exercise, you should do push-ups.

Shoulder Press

Shoulders, Triceps

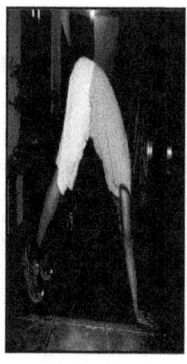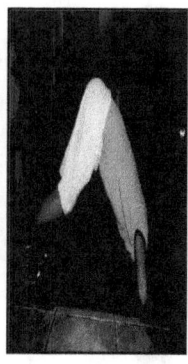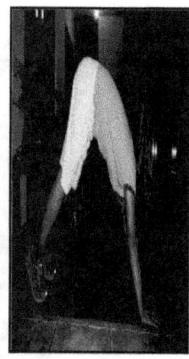

This exercise is more beneficial, if you start with your feet together. In addition, squeeze thighs together throughout the duration of the exercise.

Walk hands about six to seven hand lengths from body. Form a diamond pattern with hands. Lower your face to hands, if possible. Push up. Do what you are able to do in 30 to 60 seconds. Move slowly in order to increase strength.

Shoulder Tap Push-up

Core, Triceps, Chest

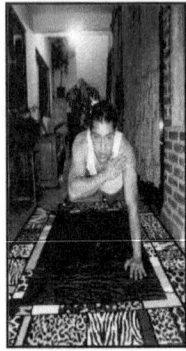 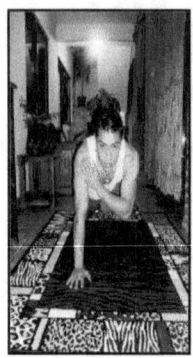 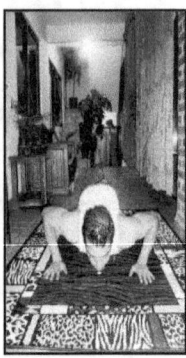 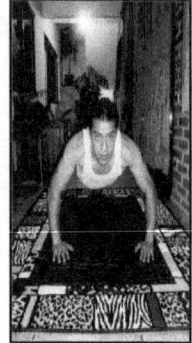

Start in the plank position. Keep core as still as possible. Raise right hand to left shoulder. Lower the right hand. Keep core as still as possible. Raise left hand to right shoulder. Return hand to floor and lower chest to floor. Return to plank position. Do this exercise for 30 to 60 seconds.

Tricep Push-up

Triceps, Core

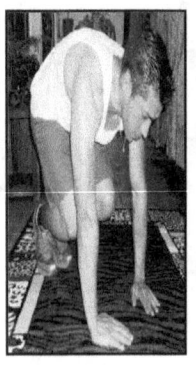 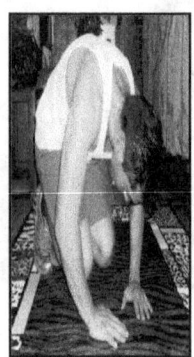

Keep feet and knees together in order to work the core. Try to maintain the arms as close to the knees as possible. Lower the shoulders and bend the arms. Do 6 repetitions and maintain proper form.

In addition to the squats and lunges typically used to strengthen the legs, the following exercises can be implemented to improve cardiovascular activity and strengthen the lungs.

Jump Squats

Calves, Thighs, Core

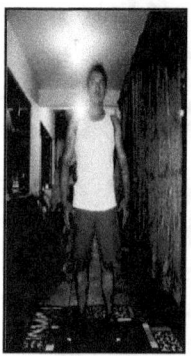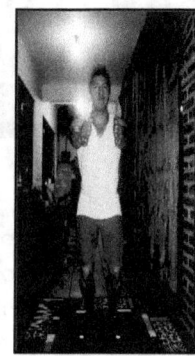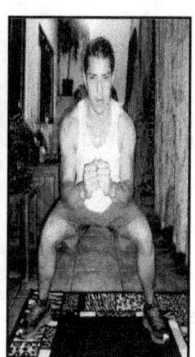

Start with hands at the side and feet together. Jump slightly and move legs so that they are more than shoulder width apart. Keep the core tight and bring arms together in front of the abdominal area. Immediately squat and jump to the starting position. Maintain a comfortable pace.

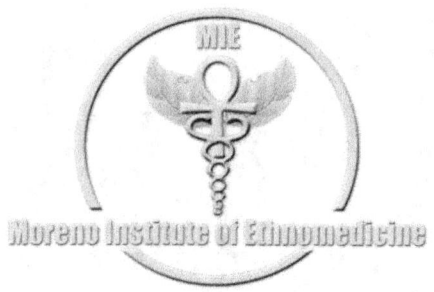

Squat & Twist

Thighs, Core, Calves

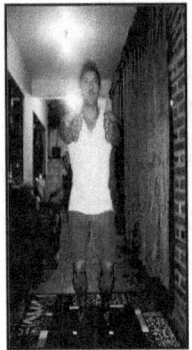 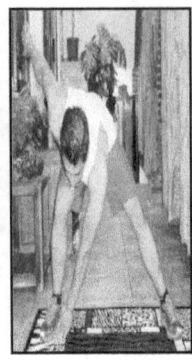 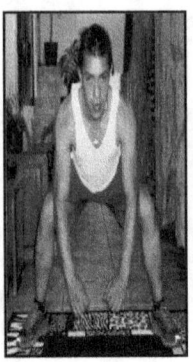 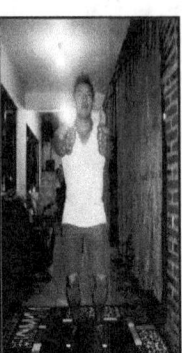

Start in standing position. Jump slightly into a squat position and reach right arm towards the opposite side of the right foot. Spring to the starting position and repeat move on the leg side with the right arm. Maintain a rhythm and pace that allows you to move for 30 to 60 seconds.

Clap & Lunge

Calves, Thighs, Shoulders and Core

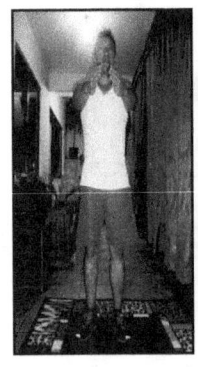 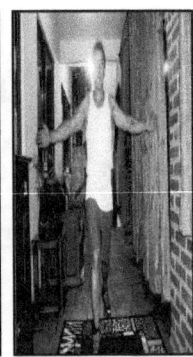 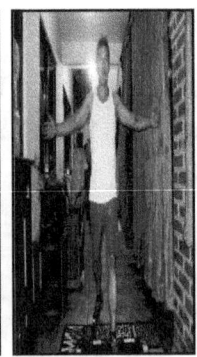 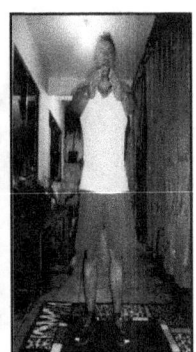

Start with the arms extended to the front and a slight bend in the knees. Do not stand erect. Maintain the arms at shoulder height throughout the exercise. Keep core tight and arms straight. Step back with left foot and move arms laterally. The lower that you are able to lower the lunge, the more you will work the thighs. Continue alternating legs for 30 to 60 seconds.

Standing Obliques

Obliques, Core, Thighs

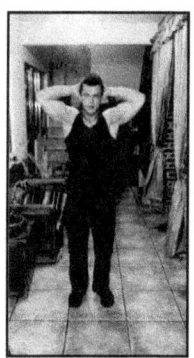 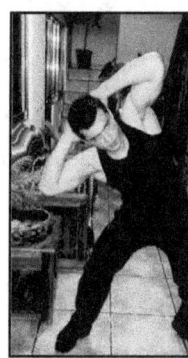 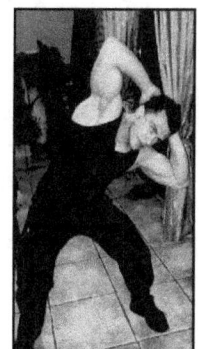

Start in a squat position with fingers interlaced and behind your head. Reach right elbow towards right thigh. Keep the core tight. Return to the center and squat and immediately reach left elbow to left thigh. Perform this exercise for 30 to 60 seconds.

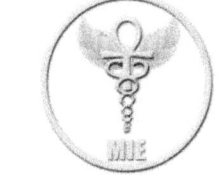

Ab Wheel

Abdominals, Shoulders, Lower Back, Core

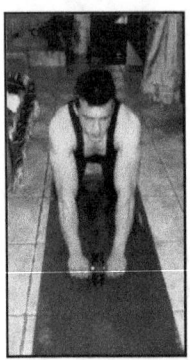 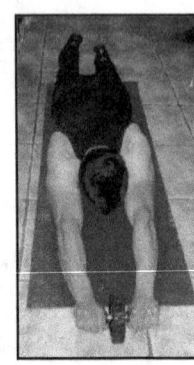 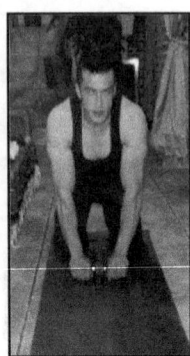

If you have an abdominal wheel, start from a kneeling position and fully extend. Keep core tight. Return to the starting position. If you do not have a wheel, use a surface in which you can slide to an extended position and back or start from the kneeling position and crawl to an extended position and walk hands back to knees.

Upward Thrust

Abdominals

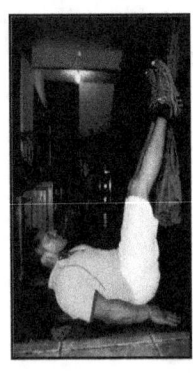 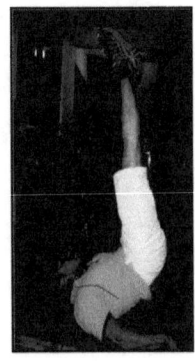

Lie on your back. If you are unable to hold your head up, you may relax it. However, by keeping your head off the floor, you will include the upper abdominals. Use your forearms to balance your body. Try not to bend your knees. Thrust legs and buttocks upward. Perform up to 25 repetitions.

Walk/Run Method is my preferred training method for quick results. If you live near a park, this is a perfect outdoor exercise. The following is a 16 minute walk/run example.

- Walk for 7 minutes
- Run for 1 minute
- Walk for 7 minutes
- Run for 1 minute - Repeat if possible.

Leg Lift

Lower Abdominals

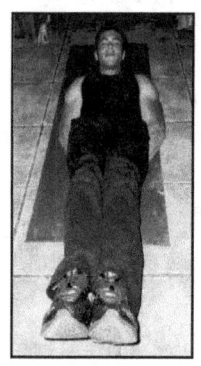 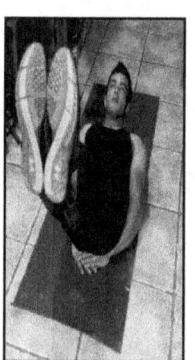

Lie on your back and place hands beneath buttocks. Head should be up in order to engage the upper abdominals. If you experience pain in the neck, keep your head on the floor. Begin with feet six inches off the floor. Lift legs to a 45 degree angle. Lower legs to the six inch mark and repeat up to 12 times at a slow pace.

Stand & Jump

Legs, Core

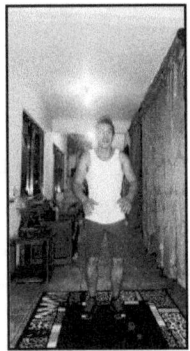 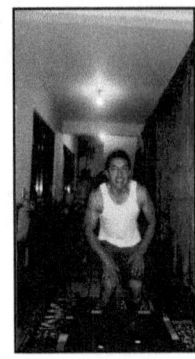 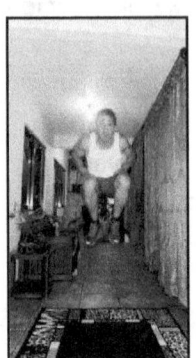

It is ideal to jump and attempt to land as softly as possible. In addition, you should bend low in order to jump from the low position. In other words, use your core and legs to jump opposed to your arms and calves.

Today, there are a number of books and DVDs about cooking and doing exercises. An advantage of the internet is the fact that several articles and videos exist on how to do yoga, calisthenics and lift weights. Unfortunately, there will continue to be such books because the majority of people have been convinced that there is an easier way to exercise and too, that anything can be eaten in moderation.

It is important that individuals undergoing exercise programs learn to vary the intensity, the number of repetitions and the *amount of rest* between the sets of exercises opposed to using a variety of exercises. Despite what you have done or have avoided doing in order to be in the state of health that you are currently suffering; you can and should make changes. More importantly, commence to remove all chemicals and over-processed foods from your life.

Ch 21 The Advantages Associated with Missing Meals

As we experience pain and illness, it is far from natural for us to contemplate changing our habits of diet. We have been conditioned by culture and society to eat. We are horrified by the idea of living life without fried, over-cooked or sweetened foods. And we never think that the drinks and foods that we consume are polluting our bodies. Some of us accept offerings of food as "love offerings" and therefore, consider the foods to be gifts from God. And if it comes from God, it is considered to be harmless. Moreover, we are convinced that "eating something" is very important. A large percentage of people think that consuming poisons in moderation is acceptable and excusable by Nature.

The addiction to food is hardly noted by persons feeding toxic bodies. Salt, sugar, preservatives, oils and bleached flours become mandatory needs as we habitually entertain the supposed hunger that has developed into an addiction due to the masking of chemicals. The human body has become a temporary recycling receptacle for chemicals. Ironically, the chemicals do damage over a period of time, for we know that cancer is not developed, felt and detected in one day. It may take years for the damage to take toll on the body as the life sustaining ability is depleted. Chemicals found in the soil, water, plants, and animals that once consumed, combine with the added chemicals in the body, and give the body a much more complicated task of determining what must be done to minimize the lethal concoctions and allow the body to function.

The idea of finding a surgery, pill or diet to prolong your youth is useless because the synthetic chemicals are aging the body and expediting the cause of deterioration. Eventually, the chemicals from the foods and medications wreak havoc on the body and a misdiagnosis is rendered. Your physician can call your symptoms anything that s/he chooses, but the chemicals are eating away the body and the act of diagnosing and prescribing drugs will only compound the problem.

Most governments are controlled by Big Business. So, having a chemical that has not been approved by a governmental agency added to food is the norm. The idea of revoking the certification or disapproving a chemical is comical because Big Business is in charge and they pretend that the chemicals have been recognized as safe. And when the body reacts to the poison, the government is trusted, Big Business is excused and the individual is made to believe that they have encountered a germ that will require surgery, medication, radiation or time to heal. Regardless, the price will be costly in some form or fashion.

Disciplined Minds

Some individuals have advanced to a level in which food is not necessary. They are elevated by life and live from the energy of atoms. They simply breathe. Perhaps, some of them wish to prolong their stay on Earth. Certainly, there is more to the concept of *breatharianism* because the monotony of sitting in one place and wishing upon a star could become just as wasteful and toxic as the behavior of persons that trust the genius of fast food restaurants to nourish their bodies. The body has been fashioned for physical activity, mental stimulation and spiritual enhancement accompanied by a fresh food method of eating. Unlike new age fanatics, African wisdom recognizes spirituality as the key to energy. Consequently, Breatharians treat the body as a temple and prove that the spirit does not need food in order to live.

Old methods of eating are mentioned regularly, due to internet, as people become bored with familiar terms and seek alternatives to the common, ineffective diets and modalities. Fruitarianism, which is not new, allows the individual to experience better health through the use of fresh, raw, uncooked foods. Life is certainly less complicated. However, once this concept becomes as commercialized as raw foodism, veganism and vegetarianism, fruits and vegetables will be grown in different soils, or waters with added nutrients, prices will increase, suitable temperatures for cooking will be argued, gadgets promising cleaner fruits will be built and no one will benefit other than the disease industry and the manufacturers of fabrications.

Half-baked scientists are already hard at work to prove that the body cannot live without cooked, processed foods. They act as if their parents magically appeared by having water added to a pill or perhaps, they arrived through the method of stork delivery. Dissuading the public is easily accomplished in the U.S. because produce is expensive and organic produce is simply uglier and more expensive.

Vitality

A spiritual relationship should exist between man and food. However, the spiritual intelligence of food is not clear because cultural perspectives, food addictions and entertainment have prevented us from understanding how our medicine is our food and how our food is our medicine. This is the reason that heat (cooking) should be avoided as much as possible. After all, the sun has properly prepared or cooked the foods for your consumption. With heat, more food is needed to provide nutrients because vitamins are susceptible to heat, light, chemicals and extreme temperature changes. By freezing foods we destroy the vitamins as well. Of course, soil conditions have already made it more difficult to get the necessary nutrients and give a feeling of satiation. Cooking further decreases the opportunity to feel "full". Vitamins are organic because they contain carbon. Of course, this gives elements with carbon and compounds (atoms of one or more elements) life. And too, vitamins are the vital minerals that are essential to the body and that energize the body.

Minerals are inorganic elements (containing atoms of the same element). Minerals are much simpler in chemical form than vitamins. Therefore, minerals are more stable to food preparation. Nonetheless, mineral loss can occur when the minerals are bound to other substances in foods and they become unavailable for utilization by the body. Again, the idea is to avoid cooked foods. Besides, food stimulates the energy that is in the body. Dead foods agitate the body and cause energy to expend. Remember, eating should not make you sleepy.

Fasting

Fasting is a good method for tuning into Nature and observing the laws of Nature. We spend a lot of time eating and/or figuring out what to eat. When we decide not to ingest food, we are bombarded with misinformation based on religious practices and/or information used to prepare for medical appointments. It is possible to do the body harm when fasting. However, fasting is not bad. It is very necessary for anyone that eats. Sick or not, an individual should fast a minimum of one 24 hour period each week. One does not have to be fanatical to get results. However, the objective is to have the desire for food suspended so that the body can be rewarded with balance. Of course, some people use fasting for spiritual enlightenment or to burn controlling desires from their bodies and minds.

Fasting is the strict act of abstaining from food. However, water is allowed during the fast. Water should be the only substance that one consumes. If juice, tea, candy, coffee, fruit or small meals are eaten (due to medication), the desire for food remains a dominant force. Fasting offers an opportunity to control the appetite. After all, over-eating contributes to kidney failure, heart disease, stroke, cancer and other illnesses because the gluttonous behavior is based on processed, dead, over-cooked foods that are incapable of offering the body the necessary nutrients.

The reason that fasting receives bad reviews is because it doesn't earn money, it isn't clearly understood and it requires sacrifice and discipline. Can it be painful and dangerous? Yes, it can be a memorable experience if the person has abused their body with sugar, cigarettes, pharmaceuticals, recreational drugs and processed foods.

The reason that fasting is considered dangerous to the disease industry is because fasting doesn't require Latin translations, drug prescriptions or costly insurance. So, to understand what most medical practitioners do not know or tell about fasting, it is imperative that we understand that fasting is going without food. Therefore, when the body is not being fed foods or toxins, it begins to purify itself and eliminate toxins. After long periods of sleep, we customarily awake with morning breath. The body has been offering signs of a toxic presence with bad breath, flatulence, and dry skin.

The body has accumulated toxins everyday of your life through breathing heavy metals and other airborne contaminants, foods, foodstuffs and medications. An individual is not likely to die in Mexico or the U.S. of starvation; malnutrition is more probable. If fasting is an issue, it is because once the fast is initiated, the body begins to dump the toxins into the bloodstream and a person is subjected to toxic dumping or toxic shock. Toxins are normally released via the urinary system and bowel movements. If this is not sufficiently accomplished, the body will use the skin. Rashes may appear; this is normal. Another source of elimination is the lungs. This is the reason for the bad breath.

Starvation occurs only after an individual has depleted the waste, fat and energy reserves that are stored in the form of glycogen. The body then begins to feed on lean tissue. This is the time when starvation becomes a concern. Otherwise, starvation is not an issue when fasting, but toxin elimination certainly is. In addition, fasting is more of a willful abstinence from food.

How Do I Know If I Need to Fast?

Not many people like to fast. A many people do not know how to fast. For individuals that avoid fasting, the body knows what it needs. Besides, the body has been doing everything possible to keep the toxins at a minimum by eliminating them, burning them in the metabolic process or storing them.

 If the stomach is distended, the body is holding toxic, decaying, dead material. Another method for determining whether fasting is needed is based on the amount of food intake versus elimination. It is possible that elimination per meal will not be achievable. However, a sizeable bowel movement should occur in the morning upon awakening even if bowel movements do not occur after every meal. Moreover, the fecal matter should float if the diet contains enough fiber.

Most persons in need of a fast will experience headaches when a meal is missed. Of course, dizziness, faintness and weakness are signs of toxicity and the individual definitely cannot fast without preparing the body through a gradual elimination of toxins.

Other factors to consider the level of toxicity are as follows:

•   Do you eat meat?

•   Do you smoke?

- Do you eat dairy products?

- Are you taking medications?

- Are you using recreational drugs?

- Do you inhale second-hand smoke regularly?

- Do you drive in congested traffic?

- Do you exercise three to five times per week?

- Do you eat cooked foods?

- Do you eat 10 to 15 pieces of fresh fruit daily?

- Do you drink 8 or more glasses of water each day?

- Do you take laxatives?

- Do you work in an industrial environment?

- Do you have lots of mucus in your body?

- Have you been diagnosed with a major disease?

Fasting is not a punishment. If the body is damaged, diseased or exhausted, it is recommended that an individual undergo a pre-fast. There is no need to increase the toxins or delay the detoxification process. It is important to drink water and eat fruit and vegetables that do not require cooking. Do not combine any foods. Eat one fruit or vegetable at a time. Wait a minimum of 30 minutes before choosing a different item to eat.

Can Anyone Fast?

Persons that have liver complications, diabetes, ulcers, kidney problems, heart disease are cautioned about fasting. In addition, persons that have been instructed by their medical doctor should consult with said physician about the matter. Matter of fact, once an individual decides to take control of his or her health; they should consult with their physician and prepare to make changes. Most doctors will not advocate fasting because its simplicity is far too complicated to be explained scientifically.

What Else Should I Know About Fasting?

It is important that the body remains hydrated. Pure water is the best. Filtered water, bottled water, spring water and well water are options, if pure water is not available. Distilled water is pure water. This can be demonstrated with a refractometer. Contrary to popular myths, alkaline water is not intended for life-time use. It should be treated as a medicinal to be used temporarily and as instructed. If one invests in a system, the water is best used for cleaning the home. Persons living in rural areas may have a means of collecting rain water; it is pure water. It is important to drink water daily, but it is more important while fasting because it assists the body in mobilizing the accumulated toxins.

Of course, elimination and enemas are important. Each day that the body abstains from food, the individual should do an enema. My preference is the enema bulb syringe because it is smaller and more appropriate considering that people have been taught to not discuss internal hygiene. And a number of people have not been instructed on the importance of assisting the colon. However, about 600ml of distilled water with the juice of a lemon is an effective solution to assist in cleansing the colon. The enema bulb is not as effective as a colonic irrigation, but it is adequate for the fast.

If the juice of a lemon is not available, use a tablespoon of organic apple vinegar or organic coffee. If coffee is used, it must be brewed. Once the solution is prepared, apply a non-petroleum substance (olive oil, avocado oil, coconut oil, etc) to the anal area for lubrication. This will facilitate the insertion of the cannula. Lie on your side. Either side is suitable due to the small amount of water. I am inclined to use the right side. Yet, some persons will argue to use the left side. And some people prefer to lie on their back. It is your choice. Once the solution has been introduced, relax and hold it for 5 to 15 minutes before expelling it. This process can be repeated.

Eating is not the answer to good health. However, eating properly is part of living properly. So, how one eats is part of the answer. As the body becomes reacquainted with cleanliness, your health will improve. Fasting does not have to be painful. It certainly should not be dangerous. If fasting threatens your health or life, you have waited too long to show appreciation for your life.

What If I Cannot Fast?

If you have a medical condition that prevents you from fasting, it is important that you take a week out of every three months to flush your body with freshly extracted juices, a fresh, raw food cleanse or a combination. This idea is effective for 2 days per week, also. During this period, do not consume any cooked, steamed, blanched or dehydrated foods. There are not any diseases that necessitate cooked food. However, some schools of thought believe that cooked food is necessary for persons with weak livers. Cooking is viewed as a process of pre-digestion. Yet, it is not necessary. If the liver is weak, it is due to eating acid forming foods such as meat, sugar, foods cooked in oil and white flour over a long period of time.

Eating one item at a time will assist in digestion. Yes, eat a fruit and wait 30 minutes to an hour. If you bore of eating a pear, orange, tomato, cucumber or avocado without combining them, or using dressings and seasonings or the wrongly suggested accompanying food groups, try extracting the juice or making a smoothie. Fruits and vegetables can be pureed for persons with weak livers and digestion problems. However, cooked food and pasteurized juices should be avoided.

Fasting has been suggested by medical authorities that recognize the relation between mind and body. It is believed that 80 percent of all illness starts in the brain. Understand that the brain's electric energy is so vital for the necessary magnetic effects in the liver; anything that alters the electric flow to the liver will alter the magnetism the same way. There are numerous things that can alter the electrical flow to the liver such as negative thoughts, cravings, depression and phobias. Again, holistically speaking, there is no separation between the mind, body and spirit.

The Mistruths about Disease

Summary

This information has been presented in an effort to encourage and enlighten the reader. It is obvious that pharmaceutical companies, egotistical scientists and physicians use fear tactics to ascertain that individuals use medications that can only cause more harm and garner more profits. And though, a percentage of people know that medications are dangerous, they chance their lives to the poisons and hope for improvement because they have accepted the medical industry as a religion, the hospital as a church and the physician as a priest. The religious is so powerful that often the physical affects are damaging.

Again, the body does not and cannot differentiate between sugar, salt, fluoride, aspartame, monosodium glutamate and the medications that are continuously being improved for marketability opposed to safety and efficacy. The body accepts and views poisons as poisons. It doesn't matter how they are shaped or colored. There are not any little, big, good or bad poisons. The body does not discriminate; they are simply poisons.

More importantly, the mind, body and spirit cannot continue to be fragmented by theory and damaging medical practices. Actually, the fragmentation is only taking place in conversation because the body is making recordings that are being projected by the mind and sometimes these messages cannot be deleted.

About the Author

Dr. Keith Moreno is a student of healthy living and ancient African wisdom. He has earned professional and doctor of philosophy degrees in Holistic Health accompanied by certifications in massage, shiatsu, colonic   irrigation, Emotional Freedom Technique, nutritional counseling, nutrition and strength conditioning, fire cupping and nutritional microscopy.

In addition to academics, Dr. Moreno has had the privilege of studying with some of America's most knowledgeable food scientists and holistic health practitioners. He has logged hundreds of hours in touch therapy, colon therapy and nutritional counseling. However, Dr. Moreno believes that his best education has been provided by persons who have trusted his knowledge while experiencing illnesses and sharing their feelings,   complaints and progress.

Dr. Moreno has an unorthodox approach to healing. As the founder of Moreno Institute of Ethnomedicine, he does not believe that any one modality is a cure-all that permits a practitioner to ignore other methods of healing. Furthermore, he feels that the physician or practitioner is not the healer, even when proven to be worthy of the title. The individual is more likely an assistant to Nature and the body that is suffering an energy loss.

He developed an interest in Reams Biological Theory of Ionization in 1996 while doing an internship in Youngstown, Ohio. Thereafter, he employed the biochemical testing techniques in his Decatur/Atlanta (Georgia) practices.

Dr. Moreno has subscribed to various forms of vegetarianism for more than three decades. Consequently, he believes that everyone is different. So, he analyzes what the body offers in its various ways before suggesting a manner of eating or correcting the abnormalities or discomforts that we refer to as disease.

Currently, Dr. Moreno relies on the analysis of blood, urine and saliva to address the ills of persons seeking his wisdom in Mexico City, Mexico. He offers global services to individuals willing to express mail biochemical samples and/or consult via Skype. In addition, he is the facilitator of holistic classes with an online academy.

References

Bibliography for The Mistruths about Disease:

- African Holistic Health by Dr. Llaila O. Afrika, Seaburn Publishing Group, 2009
- The Alcoholism and Addiction Cure by Chris Prentiss, Power Press, 2005
- Excitotoxins: The Taste That Kills by Russell L. Blaylock, M.D., Health Press, 1997
- Question Authority by James P. Hilton, Independence House Press, 2005
- Parasitic Diseases 4th Edition by Desmmier, Wadz, Hotez, Kwirsh, Apple Tree Productions, LLC, 2000
- Biologic Ionization as Applied to Human Nutrition by Dr. A.F. Beddoe, S&J Unlimited, 1994
- Melanin by Dr. Llaila O. Afrika, Seaburn Publishing, 2009
- What Your Doctor Doesn't Know About Nutritional Medicine May Be Killing You by Ray D. Strand, M.D., Thomas Nelson Publishers, 2002
- PH Madness by Roger Bezanis, Neff/Harris Publishing, 2010
- Race and Human Evoluton by Milford Wolpoff and Rachel Caspari, Westview Press, 1997
- Signs and Symptoms Analysis From A Functional Perspectiveby Dicken Weatherby, N.D., Nutritional Therapy Association, 2004
- Diagnostic Medical Parasitology by Lynne, Shore, Garcia, ASM Press, 2007
- Nutricide by Dr. Llaila O. Afrika, Seaburn Publishing Group, 2009
- Tissue Cleansing Through Bowel Management by Bernard Jensen, D.C., Bernard Jensen Enterprises, 1981
- The African Background to Medical Science by Charles S. Finch, Red Sea Press, 1990

3-Words!

3 Words

Control Your Life!

3-Words

Stand Between
You & Your Goals.

Discover Your

3-Words.

http://www.My3Words.org

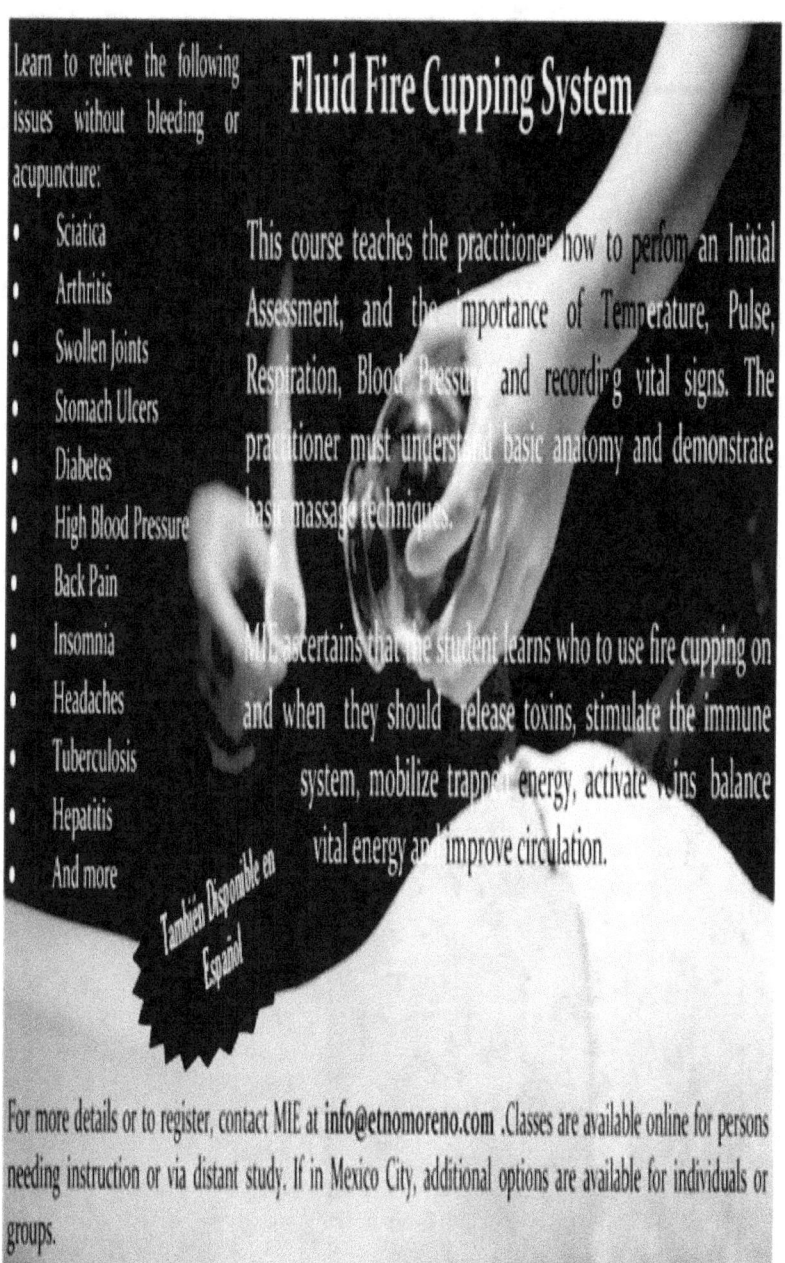

Learn to relieve the following issues without bleeding or acupuncture:

- Sciatica
- Arthritis
- Swollen Joints
- Stomach Ulcers
- Diabetes
- High Blood Pressure
- Back Pain
- Insomnia
- Headaches
- Tuberculosis
- Hepatitis
- And more

Tambien Disponible en Espanol

Fluid Fire Cupping System

This course teaches the practitioner how to perform an Initial Assessment, and the importance of Temperature, Pulse, Respiration, Blood Pressure and recording vital signs. The practitioner must understand basic anatomy and demonstrate basic massage techniques.

MIE ascertains that the student learns who to use fire cupping on and when they should release toxins, stimulate the immune system, mobilize trapped energy, activate veins balance vital energy and improve circulation.

For more details or to register, contact MIE at **info@etnomoreno.com** .Classes are available online for persons needing instruction or via distant study. If in Mexico City, additional options are available for individuals or groups.

143

DRIED BLOOD ANALYSIS
Course
(El Curso de Análisis de Sangre Seca)

Become a Nutritional Microscopist!

The course focuses on dried blood samples and familiarizes the analyst with live cells, as well. The analyst will have adequate knowledge to start seeing clients upon completion of the course.

- Learn how to properly take dried blood samples.
- Identify the causes of disease.
- Offer Nutritional Recommendations and Lifestyle Solutions.
- Identify blood indicators and how they influence the client's health.
- Clarify the controversial alkaline/acid balance.
- Learn how to function in business as a Nutritional Microscopist.

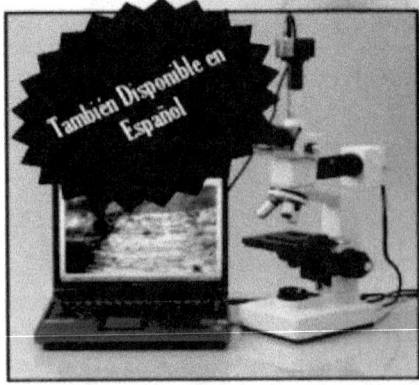

Available online via distance study or virtual classroom.

Class can be taken without microscope.

Classes available for groups at your location.

For details contact MIE at info@etnomoreno.com

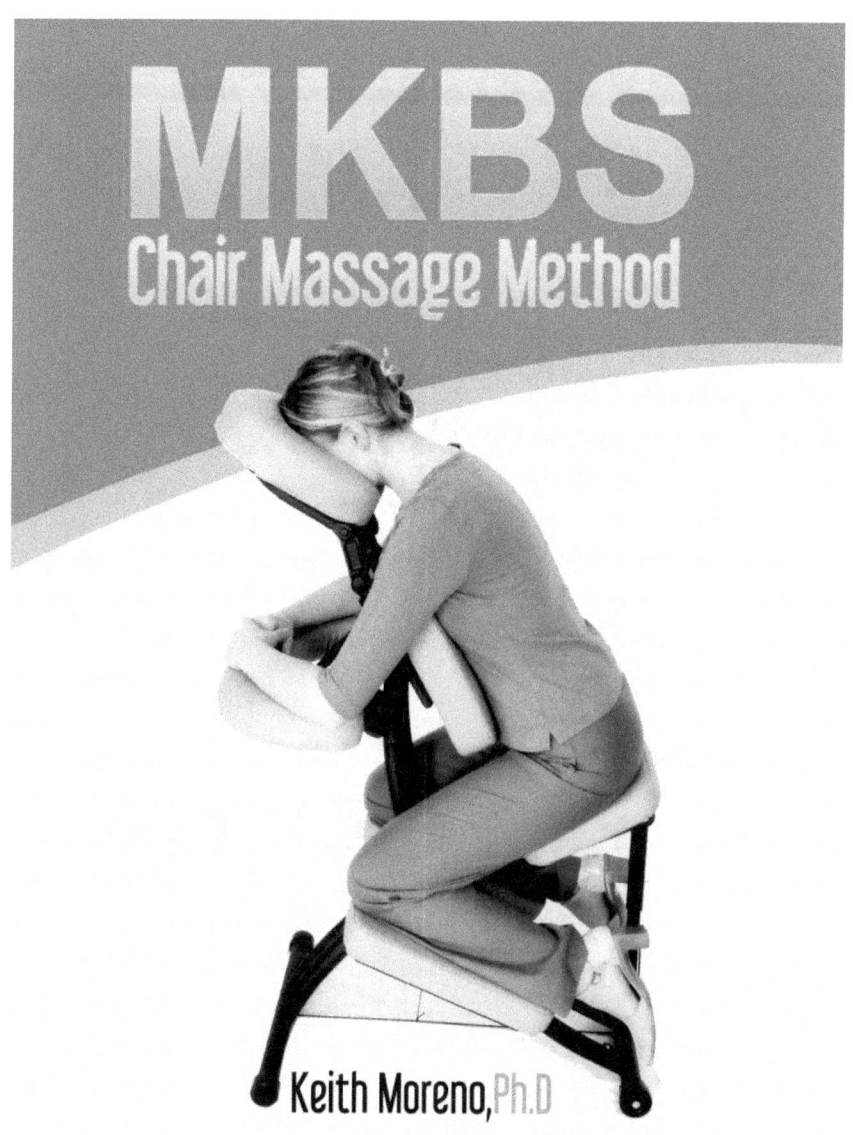

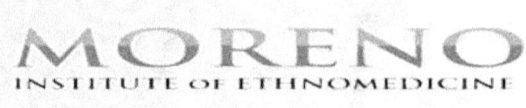

- COMPREHENSION & UTILIZATION OF VITAL SIGNS

- NUTRITIONAL MICROSCOPY: DRY BLOOD ANALYSIS

- BIOCHEMICAL ANALYSIS

- FIRE CUPPING MASSAGE

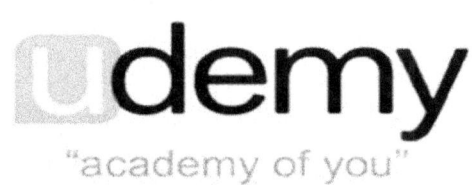

"academy of you"

The Mistruths about Disease